M000278396

Healthy by Design

Weight Loss, God's Way

The Proven 21-Day Weight Loss Devotional Bible Study

Cathy Morenzie

Guiding Light Publishing

First Edition: July 2008

Second Edition: January 2011

Third Edition: December 2013

Fourth Edition: April 2015

Fifth Edition: September 2019

ISBN: 978-0-9958443-8-4 (print)

978-0-9958443-9-1 (digital)

Published by Guiding Light Publishing
261 Oakwood Avenue, York, ON, Canada, M63 2V3

Note: The information in this book is for educational purposes only and is not recommended as a means of diagnosing or treating illness. All situations concerning physical or mental health should be supervised by a health professional knowledgeable in treating that particular condition. Neither the author nor anyone affiliated with Healthy by Design dispenses medical advice, nor do they prescribe any remedies or assume any responsibility for anyone who chooses to treat themselves.

Cover Design by: kimmontefortedesign.com

Cover & author photos by http://www.martinbrownphotography.ca/

Interior Design by: Davor Dramikanin

Table of Contents

A Note From the Author

You're about to change your life! As you embark on this health and faith journey, I couldn't be more excited for you and honored to encourage you along the path.

Every day, people like you share how our *Healthy by Design* books and *Weight Loss, God's Way* online programs have transformed their lives, from reaching their weight goals to increasing their sense of worthiness and self-confidence, while also deepening their relationship with their Heavenly Father.

This book is the start of your journey, but if you want to ultimately reach your goal weight and maintain it you need to continue building on the foundations presented in this book. To help you carry on I've created these special resources for you, so you can experience faster results and maintain them permanently.

QUICK-START TOOLKIT: Our FREE gift to you for having purchased this book. The toolkit includes the following:

- Printable .pdf workbook
- Quick-Start Checklist
- Sample 7-Day Meal Plan
- Low-Impact Workout Video

- 3 Steps of Overcoming Emotional Eating Guide
- Faith-based weight loss insights, tips, and special offers in our bi-weekly email devotional

www.weightlossgodswaybonus.com

Praying for your Success,

Cathy Morenzie

www.cathymorenzie.com

FOREWARD

Like many of us my journey of health, fitness, and attempting to achieve and maintain a healthy weight has been similar to a roller coaster ride. Plenty of ups, downs, and unexpected curves, which can leave your head (and heart) spinning. There were times when I couldn't wait to step on the scale, and times when, well, let's just say it fell into the 'not so pleasant' category.

Without a doubt, the greatest success that I have had on a long-term, consistent basis was when working in partnership with Cathy Morenzie. Her God-given, cut to the chase, common sense approach to training, nutrition, and balance has been an emotional and practical inspiration to me again and again. From writing down my goals, journaling my food intake, committing it all to God, to keeping the long-term goals in mind, I have developed into not only a goal-setter but a goal-getter! You can also add six-time marathoner to that!

Praise the Lord! Cathy has decided to share her learning and experience from the Lord with not only with her clients but with us as well. In *Healthy by Design—Weight Loss, God's Way*, she has compiled the wisdom she has gleaned from over 30 years of being a personal trainer, and we stand to benefit immensely if we take it to heart.

Whatever your goal is (or goals are)—a number on a scale; that look of satisfaction in what you see in the mirror; fitting comfortably into a new or favorite outfit; honoring God with your eating habits; and/or maybe even crossing a finish line, I want to encourage you that you can do it. And there is assistance to be had! Using the book in your hands you can see these dreams come to fruition, and you will be blessed as a result.

On the faith and fitness journey,

Herbie Kuhn

Professional Sports Chaplain, Basketball Announcer, and Impact Speaker

INTRODUCTION

The Problem

Do you have any idea how powerful you are? Have you ever thought about it? In Luke 10:19, Jesus says, *"I have given you authority to trample on snakes and scorpions and to overcome all the power of the enemy; nothing will harm you."* And that's just one of many scriptures that talk about the power we have in Christ.

So if we have all this power and authority, why do we feel so powerless? How is it that we have been given the power and authority to cast out demons, yet we can't stop ourselves from eating a piece of chocolate? Why do we struggle with so many issues around our weight, such as emotional eating, physical inactivity, self-control, guilt, and feelings of low self-esteem?

A 2006 Purdue University study by Ken Ferraro, and later a 2011 Northwestern University study by Matthew Feinstein, discovered that religious Americans were more likely to be overweight than their nonreligious peers. How can this be? Shouldn't we be the healthiest people on the planet because of the promises that God has given us? Where's the disconnect? The Purdue study indicated that many of the factors related to being overweight were associated with the increased social activities churchgoers participated in—such as after-church brunches and get-togethers. The fellowshipping with our fellow brothers and sisters is nice, but we need solutions to this health crisis. We don't need another church dinner, bake sale, or barbecue.

The problem is analogous to an air conditioner on a scorching hot day. We have been given an indispensable tool to help us, but until we plug in the air conditioner we will never receive the benefits and the power that exist at our disposal. Until we call on the Holy Spirit to be our helper, as our instruction book tells us, we will never walk in the authority we have been given.

The Program

Healthy by Design: Weight Loss, God's Way is just one of a series of books and programs I've written to help women discover the missing steps that have been blocking their weight loss success.

This book is a 21-day devotional bible study and challenge that will take you through the key habits, mindsets, and behaviors of weightreleasing based on biblical principles. To get the maximum benefit from the program you should carve out at least 20 minutes per day to complete the daily action steps, and take time throughout your day to reflect on the scripture. At the end of the day, you should read it again and record your thoughts based on that topic.

The Daily Messages

Each daily message portrays a character from the Bible to teach us that our challenges are not unique; God understands them and wants to help us if we allow Him. They also teach us how faith plays an integral part in our lives and our victory.

The Daily Health Challenges

We believe that you have to challenge yourself if you truly want to change. Nothing has ever happened from the comfort of your couch. Stepping out of your comfort zone and trusting God to help you achieve your health goals will radically transform your health and your faith.

The daily health challenges will inspire you to put your faith into action. They are designed to have you rethink how you've been approaching your weight loss journey. They are designed to viscerally take you out of your habitual patterns and behaviors and allow the Holy Spirit to show you healthier ways of thinking and behaving. To get the most out of the challenges, put in the time to do them and let your results speak for themselves!

The Practice Habits

In addition to the daily challenges, I also encourage you to make one small change in your daily health habits. Too often people try to change too much and end up overwhelmed. As you start the 21-days, commit to practicing one of the following actions:

1. Commit to exercising every day for a minimum of 15 minutes.
2. Commit to tracking everything you eat using MyFitnessPal or another online app of your choice.
3. Commit to not eating anything after 7:00 pm (or three hours before bed).

The Daily Confessions

The daily confessions provide an opportunity to speak God's Word back to Him. They are all based on scripture and will help to change your thought patterns about your health, your weight, and your life in general.

An appendix is located at the back of the book, where you can study and meditate at your leisure on a particular area that might be a stronghold for you.

Continue for 21 days straight, including weekends. If you skipped a day or had a day you didn't initially gain insight from, don't worry—take as much time as you need on each chapter.

The Preparation

How are you feeling right now? You may be apprehensive or excited, or perhaps have a fear of failing ... again. In the course of this program, you may go through a roller-coaster ride of emotions. I encourage you to keep a journal handy to write out any feelings that may come to the surface. Ask the Holy Spirit to reveal new truths and insights to you and to gently change you.

Throughout this book avoid the tendency to judge yourself, your actions, or your choices. There will be no right or wrong; no guilt or condemnation (Rom. 8:1). Just notice what comes up for you and invite the Holy Spirit to make you present to your feelings; to show you the root of your stronghold(s) (Ps. 139:23-24); and to gird you for the journey.

Here's how you can prepare for the daily habit challenge:

If you're choosing exercise as your goal ...

- What type of exercise do you plan to do?
- What time of the day will you do it?
- Do you have the right shoes, equipment, etc.?

- Ask yourself, what are some challenges that might get in your way? How can you remedy them?

If you're tracking your food ...

- Have you downloaded the MyFitnessPal app yet?
- What foods will you need to purchase or give up to stay within your calories?
- Will you track as you eat or at the end of the day?

If you're committing to not eating after 7:00 pm ...

- When will you prepare your meals?
- Are you home late any evenings?
- Do you have any evening commitments?

These challenges are suggestions so feel free to choose one of your own.

Bottom line, avoid the urge to try to suddenly eat in a dramatically different way. Remember that there are no quick fixes to anything. Change is a process. You will learn that "trying" is rarely successful. Flesh can't change flesh, but the Holy Spirit can help you if you will let Him. He is ready and available to you 24/7 if you call on Him.

Are you familiar with the expression "Sow where you want to go"? It means that you should begin to do the action that you want to see manifested in your own life.

Begin to pray for other people also going through this process, and know that they will be praying for you.

The Process

The goal of this program is to promote permanent change through a series of small doable incremental changes. Baby steps if you will.

This plan will run for 21 consecutive days, but note that 21 days is only a suggestion. You may choose to read this plan and scripture every other day. Also, remember that this is only the beginning. You are on a life-long journey!

Each day you will read the weight loss principle, recite the daily confession, and follow through on the daily action step. Remember, there are no quick fixes. You simply must put in the time to allow growth and change to take place.

Please understand that this is not a book to teach you about exercises or foods that will help you lose weight. I'm willing to bet that you already know about these things. Instead, you will learn the patterns, behaviors, and mind-sets that keep you stuck in the same cycle of gaining and losing weight, along with the ageless biblical principles to overcome those mindsets that have kept you in bondage.

The Principles

God has given us immutable laws and principles to govern our lives. These principles apply to every person, every situation, and every circumstance. Even if you do not practice them per se, you will still experience the consequences if you go against them. Use these principles in your weight releasing journey and other areas of your life to experience the victory, freedom, and peace that God has already given you.

God wants to transform our lives little by little. Weight releasing is a process! (2 Cor. 3:18)

There's nothing inspiring or motivating about the thought of slow and steady—especially when it comes to weight loss.

Though it may have taken us years to gain weight, we want to lose it fast. However, to be successful, we must understand that losing weight is a process. It will not happen overnight, and we must gird ourselves to understand that the process will take time. 2 Corinthians 3:18 teaches us that God's glory comes in levels or stages when we partner with the Lord's Spirit.

Though there are many instantaneous miracles that happen in the Bible, you should understand that the qualities that God needs to develop in you to make your weight loss permanent will not happen miraculously. They need to be rehearsed and become ingrained in your subconscious mind. As frustrating as it may seem, it will take some time. But know that God has given you the capacity to be patient in the process once you submit the process to Him.

Understand that, though the process may seem slow, the Word tells us that God is not slow in fulfilling His promises (2 Pet. 3:9). God will work in tandem with your obedience, so get ready to receive what He has for you right away!

God wants us to partner with the Holy Spirit to live a victorious life. (John 14:15-25)

In this scripture, Jesus tells his disciples that God will send the Holy Spirit who will live with us and be with us always. He will guide us and be our advocate and helper. If you've tried to release weight on your own then you know that it can be a frustrating process, often with more failures than successes. Now imagine letting go of all the anxiety and frustration, no longer living by letting the number on the scale determine the type of mood you will be in.

Imagine the confidence and peace you will feel at a social function. God's rich promises can all be yours when you allow the Holy Spirit to partner with you in this and every other stronghold in your life.

God has provided us with choices, and He wants us to choose the best way. (Deut. 30:19)

Action/Consequences: From Adam and Eve to Revelation, God gives us the choice between right and wrong, blessings and curses. God created us with free will and would never impose His will on us. He lets us decide the choices we will make in life. Through our choices, we learn wisdom and understanding.

Though it's not always obvious, many of the choices we make will bring blessings or curses. Choosing to sleep in, have an extra slice of cake, or skip another workout are not curses in and of themselves, but they will weaken your discipline muscle which will eventually lead to poor health.

Conversely, and fortunately, taking the time to eat a proper breakfast, minimizing your intake of coffee, processed foods and sugar, and exercising regularly will not miraculously bring blessings to your life, but will help you feel better. All these things will increase your energy and your mood, and help you manage your weight and build your self-esteem, which will have many long-term blessings.

It may seem daunting right now, but rest assured that God will teach you how to make good choices that will richly bless your life.

God wants to use our good health to glorify Him and to be an example to others. (1 Cor. 6:19-20)

God dwells in our physical bodies and calls it His temple. A temple is a sacred place of beauty and majesty. God took great pride and joy in creating us, and He also wants us to treat our bodies as the sacred temples He designed them to be.

We've all looked at other people and wondered how they could be Christians when they (insert a vice here). Although God Himself is not judging or condemning you, you probably know within yourself that you're not being as effective as you want to be because your weight is getting in the way.

You know that you would have more confidence, energy, stamina, and effective witnessing when you are living at the level of health that God created you to live in.

Since writing the first edition of this book in 2008 and growing in the Lord, the Holy Spirit has led me to five more biblical principles that you can apply to your health journey. As you study the scriptures, see how they apply to you.

1. Identification: Good health is your identity, not your destination. Gen. 1:27

You were created to be in good health—after all, you were created in God's image. Think about that for a minute ... you were created in God's image!

The bible says, "*Then God said, 'Let Us make man in Our image, according to Our likeness; and let them rule over the fish of the sea and over the birds of the sky and over the cattle and over all the earth, and over every creeping thing that creeps on the earth.' God created man in His own image, in the image of God He created him; male and female He created them.* (Genesis 1:26-27 NASB)

So if that's true, then why have you spent so many years of your adult life trying to get to a specific number on the scale? Just think about the wasted energy, time, frustration, and happiness you've lost trying to achieve something you already possess.

Soooooo the message here is to:

Stop trying so hard to work at something you already possess. Focus on trusting God more and trying less.

Stop being afraid of success. Success is in your DNA—it's *who you are!*

Stop chasing a mythical, magical illusion of what you think your life would look like at a certain weight. It's time to see and accept the awesomeness of who you are right now. Without acceptance, it will be difficult if not impossible to make progress.

Stop waiting, wishing, wanting, hoping, praying, and wasting time worrying about the future. God is a right now God; He is here in the present, guiding you step by step.

I know, easier said than done. But as you begin to trust that good health is part of your identity, then you will stop wasting so much time searching for a magical, mythical fantasy that doesn't exist and begin to embrace who God has called you to be—regardless of your current size.

2. Ternion (triad): Good health involves a combination of healing your body, soul, and spirit. 1 Thess. 5:23

God made us distinct and unique from all of creation.

Because we were created in God's image, He also created us with a tripartite nature like himself. As God encompasses the Father, Son and Holy Spirit, we too are also composed of three parts. Our spirit, soul, and body.

As human beings we live in a physical body, we have a soul, and we live eternally as a spirit that connects with God's spirit. Our tripartite nature works to keep us healthy and whole. It's impossible to address one area without giving attention to the other.

The bible says, *"Now may the God of peace Himself sanctify you entirely; and may your spirit and soul and body be preserved complete, without blame at the coming of our Lord Jesus Christ"* (1 Thessalonians 5:23 NASB).

For us to be in total health as God intended, all three parts of our being need to be healthy.

They are intertwined and interconnected. Here's how:

Body

Our body is our outer shell, but it houses the temple of the living God. It is your physical being. It consists of our five senses: taste, touch, sight, smelling, and hearing. In His infinite wisdom, God created our bodies to operate in harmony with our souls and spirits. If our physical bodies are not healthy, it negatively impacts our spirits and our souls.

Here's what the bible teaches us about our physical bodies:

It houses the living God (1Cor 3:16-17).

We are to present it to God as a living sacrifice (Romans 12:2).

We are to put no confidence in it (Phil 3:3).

We are to discipline it and keep it under control (1 Cor 9:27).

Soul

Our souls are made up of our conscious and our subconscious minds, which house our thoughts, conscience, will, and emotions. It gives us our personality. This is where the battle rages. It's where we experience the anxiety, doubts, and fears which manifest in our bodies as excess weight and illness. If our soul is bound then we will have difficulty honoring our temples, and we will have difficulty connecting with God.

Here's what the bible teaches us about our souls:

The Lord created in us a living soul (Gen 2:7).

It is immortal (Matt 10:28).

It is in conflict with our spirit (1 Cor 2:14).

They can lead us away and lead to sin and death (James 1:13-15).

Spirit

At our core is our spirit, it's the part of us that connects with God. This is our contact point with God where our spirit communicates with His. Paul says, "When we cry 'Abba! Father' it's the spirit himself bearing witness with our spirit that we are children of God." (Romans 8:15-17.) It's only when we align our spirits with our Heavenly Father's, that we be ever be successful at anything we do, including getting healthier.

Here's what the bible teaches us about our spirits:

God enlightens our spirit so we can know truth (Proverbs 20:27).

The indwelling Spirit of Christ dwells in our heart (Romans 8:16).

God's Word can divide our soul and spirit (Heb 4:12).

Key takeaway: We are tripartite beings. Whatever happens to one part of our being has repercussions in the other two areas.

3. Revelation: Information without revelation is meaningless. (Rom 8:5, Rom 12:2, James 1:5)

Here's an obvious, but important, question. Do you need more information on weight loss? Didn't think so. You probably already have more information than you can ever read. The problem is not a lack of information but the exact opposite. Most of us suffer from information overload. You probably have books sitting on your bookshelf or table that you mean to read, emails that you need to respond to, interesting articles that you one day hope to skim.

Most women I talk to are so overwhelmed that I know for sure that the answer you're looking for isn't found in reading another book or signing up for another program.

Information in and of itself is meaningless. Ask yourself the following questions about all the information you've gathered to date.

Revelation comes from the Holy Spirit. It doesn't come from our wisdom or intellect. In fact, it's our intellect that keeps getting us into trouble. We 'think' we know more than God, so we keep taking matters back into our own hands. James 1:5 reminds us that it is God who gives us wisdom.

1. Are you applying it?

What good is it to say you trust God with your health yet never submit the journey to Him or never run to Him in your time of need? It's one thing to read something in the Bible or even in a book, but without relying on the power of the Holy Spirit to transform us it's just information, which has no power on its own. Remember this: Knowledge is NOT power; application of knowledge is power.

2. Have you mastered it?

I remember singing up for one of those online 30-day squat challenges. I got up to day four and I quit. Yet if someone asked me, I would probably say, "Yeah, I've done it before." That's what many of us do. We invest in something and quit before we've achieved results, yet we talk like we're now experts on the subject.

I have a similar challenge with tracking my food. Yes, I track it, but am I using the tool effectively to eat within my daily allowance or use it as an effective tool for weight-management? The answer is no, so until then I will continue using it until I learn what I need to learn from the tool. Don't get frustrated or give up if you miss a few days or if you can't stick to it. Keep on trying until you master it.

3. Do your results prove it?

This is the biggest test of true knowledge. I remember striking up a conversation with this marketing 'guru' who began telling me about a new miracle fat-loss pill that has been selling like hotcakes. He told me all the benefits of the product and how amazing it was, and was about 50 pounds overweight! Or have you ever had the sister at church tell you a Word of the Lord for you, yet her life was in shambles?

Let your results speak louder than your words. Results never lie. If you're not getting results in your weight-loss program, stop wasting time gathering more useless information.

4. Transformation: Transformation comes through daily submission. (2 Cor 10:5, Luke 9:23)

Let's face it, sacrificing anything isn't pleasant at the time. Even the word itself conjures up feelings of pain and struggle. Yet our Bible teaches us that living a life of sacrifice is the only way to enjoy a life of freedom in Christ. In Matthew 10:39 Jesus says, "Whoever finds his life will lose it, and whoever loses his life for my sake will find it."

The reality is that many of us are frustrated and feel utterly hopeless with our current state of health, but are unwilling to make the necessary sacrifices it takes to achieve a healthy weight. We've been struggling with our weight for most of our lives and it feels like things will never change. Despite our feelings of hopelessness, we keep grasping at short-term worldly solutions to end our pain. We keep trying solution after solution, but they eventually get too difficult, time-consuming, or we just get bored and move on to the next thing.

It's only when we can embrace Jesus' teaching that short-term sacrifice will lead to long-term fulfillment, and the concept of sacrificial living will not be so daunting.

The solution is found in God. Until we know the true heart of God, sacrifice will always seem like deprivation or punishment, but it's the exact opposite. Freedom is found in dying to ourselves every hour of every day so that we can live an abundant life.

1. God calls us to submission because He understands how easily we are led away by our flesh if we don't exercise restraint. He knows our propensity to make idols out of everything and how these idols will turn our attention away from Him.

> *"No one can serve two masters. Either you will hate the one and love the other, or you will be devoted to the one and despise the other. You cannot serve both God and money."* Matthew 6:24

2. God calls us to submission because He knows that our insatiable desires for food (money, power, sex) will always keep us wanting even more. We try to fill our needs with worldly things instead of Godly things, so no matter how much food we

eat we will always want more. No matter how much money we make we will always want more (or whatever your weakness is).

"But each one is tempted when he is carried away and enticed by his own lust. Then when lust has conceived, it gives birth to sin; and when sin is accomplished, it brings forth death..." James 1:14-15

3. God calls us to submission because He knows that He is the only one who can fulfill all of our needs. When we sacrifice our appetites and draw closer to God He honors our actions, meets us in our time of need, and draws closer to us. Satiety and satisfaction are found in Him alone.

"Blessed are those who hunger and thirst for righteousness, for they will be filled." Matthew 5:6

As you read this book you begin to embrace your health journey as a marathon, not a sprint. You will realize the futility of searching for the quick fixes and easy answers and finally grasp that there is no such thing.

You simply can't cram what the Holy Spirit is trying to teach you on this journey. It's not like a high school test. You're on the journey of your life and it will take time and patience.

Change is a daily process. It's the little things that you do daily that will get you to your goals.

Every time you say 'yes' to God, you will move closer to your goal.

5. Action: You must move past the natural resistance from contemplation to action. (Jas 1:22; Jas 2:26)

What do I mean by natural resistance?

Resistance refers to the trials, roadblocks, difficulties, frustrations, set-backs, and hinderances you encounter on your journey. It could be anything from backsliding, self-sabotage, an injury, an illness in the family, traveling, vacation, family visiting, unexpected company, or anything that slows down or stops your weight loss. Some of this resistance is God perfecting us, some is the enemy trying to keep us from fulfilling God's promises for us, and some is the results of our faulty thinking and poor choices. Wherever the resistance comes from, we all must move through it.

When we experience resistance, most of us usually do one of two things: We either dig our heels in deeper or we quit. What if I told you that neither of these options were correct? Resistance is not to be fought. Think of quicksand—the more you resist, the faster you sink. The resistance is to be released to God so that we can 'cast our cares on Him' as we find the courage to take action. Instead of always 'getting ready to get ready', planning to start your new diet on 'Monday', or doing more research on the right program for you— stop procrastinating and take action already. That's what this last principle means and that's what you'll begin to discover how to do.

The Purpose

Americans spend $66 billion a year on weight loss programs and products. You probably have spent hundreds, if not thousands yourself, on products or programs promising you fast results.

You need a solution for how to release the weight without falling for sales gimmicks and unhealthy diets. What if I told you that you never had to spend another penny on a weight loss gimmick? This book was written to help you achieve the best health of your life, as well as to draw you closer to God. God doesn't want you going around the same mountain, time and time again. He wants you free. 2 Corinthians 3:17 says, *"Where the spirit of the Lord is, there is liberty".* Beloved, I want you to experience that liberty.

For more than half of my life, I tried to change just about everything about myself. I felt I was too fat, too hippy, too loud, too soft-spoken, too ugly, too conservative, too black, too easy, too afraid, too lazy, too worldly, too Godly, and most of all, too undisciplined to make any of these changes stick. Talk about bondage!

Not until I cried out like Paul did in Romans 7:24 to be delivered from this body of death, did I begin to receive God's healing, peace, and rest from all the stories I was telling myself. It's an incredible feeling of rest to be able to do less and receive more. My prayer is that you will receive the same.

The process of God gently changing me continues day by day—bit by bit. I want to share with you what God has taught me so far. I pray that you receive it and allow it to shape you into the precious miracle that God has created you to be.

I love you and pray for your victory.

Cathy Morenzie

21 DAYS GOD'S WAY

Day 1
WHAT'S YOUR GOAL?

Scripture Reflection

"The plans of the diligent lead to profit as surely as haste leads to poverty." (Proverbs 21:5 NIV)

"Failing to plan, is planning to fail."
~ Benjamin Franklin

So you're ready to start your weight loss journey. Congratulations! Before you can start, do you know what you want? Do you know how long it will take you to reach your goal? Your goal will begin to come to fruition only when you are clear on what you want. Writing down your goal sends out a clear message to yourself and the world about who you are and what you are capable of completing. Day 1 will be the most time-consuming but crucial step in the entire plan. Knowing what you want is crucial to getting to where you're going. After all, if you don't know your goal aside from just saying you want to lose weight, there are hundreds of programs out there ready to lead you down the frustrating, never-ending path of weight loss.

As you write down your goals, you will begin to align your will with your heavenly Father's. To become crystal clear on your goals they must be specific, measurable, attainable, realistic, and time-constrained (S.M.A.R.T.). To learn all about

SMART goal setting, go the appendix at the end of this book. Here is a brief summary.

SPECIFIC.

Be specific about the results you want and what you will do to achieve the goal. Instead of saying "I want to lose weight", choose a specific number.

MEASURABLE.

Can you tangibly show how you will meet your goal? What are the objective markers along the way that will confirm that you are moving in the right direction?

You must be able to track your progress to make sure you are on the right track

ATTAINABLE.

Get clear on what is and is not possible for you.

REALISTIC AND RELEVANT.

In order to set realistic goals, you will develop an understanding of just what it takes to release weight. Most of our goals are unrealistic because we don't understand the process of weight loss. Are your goals in line with your Christian values and possible based on your current lifestyle?

TIME-CONSTRAINED.

Time-constrained goals mean that your goal should have a start date and an end date. The amount of time that you give yourself to attain your goal should create a sense of urgency, yet should also be realistic enough that it is possible to achieve it.

It's highly likely that you've set goals many times before and have had limited levels of success. So why will it be different this time? In Luke 14:28-30 we learn that you would never consider building a house without estimating the costs, the time, and all the factors involved in the project. And you would never attempt to start a weight releasing program without having specific indices to measure your success.

Today's Health Challenge

Follow this example to write out your goal using the SMART principle. 9.19.22

I (insert name) Janine commit to 144.5 releasing (insert weight) 10 pounds/kgs./stone by (insert date) NOV. 14. I will do this by (insert action steps) eating healthy, cutting sweets, drinking water, walking 4 times a week.

Additional Study

1. Meditate on the scripture, *"Suppose one of you wants to build a tower. Won't you first sit down and estimate the cost to see if you have enough money to complete it?"* (Luke 14:28 NIV) What is the Holy Spirit showing you about the importance of planning and goal setting?

2. Reflect on how you've gone about trying to achieve your goals in the past. Have you applied the principles in Luke 14:28? If not, will you commit to this process?

3. Commit this journey to God and ask Him to help you set Godly goals that will glorify Him.

Today's Confession

Thank You for giving me the wisdom to set realistic goals that glorify You. I submit my goals and plans to You and trust You to show me the way to bring my goals into alignment with Your will and purpose for my life. I declare that my goals will come to fruition. I am successful and victorious in the name of Jesus.

Workspace/Reflections

smaller portions at dinner - no 2nd's

no candy, cookies, sweets after dinner

2 desserts on weekends

pizza - once a week - 2 slices

Day 2

COUNT THE COST: WHAT ARE YOU WILLING TO DO?

Scripture Reflection

"Then Jesus said to his disciples, 'If anyone would come after me...'" (Matthew 16:24 NLT)

"Something happens whenever you sacrifice."
~ T.D. Jakes

There's no denying that there are mindset differences between thin and healthy people vs. people who struggle to maintain their weight. Thin people see food, their health, their bodies, exercise, and life in general from a different perspective than overweight people. They make definite and distinct CHOICES and are willing to make sacrifices that most others don't. So the real question for the person trying to lose weight becomes, "How much are you willing to do?" If weight release is something you really want, then get ready to make the necessary changes to make it happen.

- Are you willing to make the time for exercise regardless of how you feel?
- Are you willing to eat only when you're hungry and stop when you're full?
- Are you willing to eat for health and not for pleasure?

- Are you willing to pay the price?
- Are you willing to accept that you are 100 percent responsible for your weight release?
- Are you willing to go for counseling or commit to additional support that you might need to overcome your blockages?

The famous 'Faith Hall of Fame' in Hebrews 11 is a perfect example of people in the Bible who overcame the odds and pushed past their comfort level to do what they were called to do. Noah subjected himself to the ridicule of his entire community to build a huge boat on dry land (Gen. 6:1–11:32). At God's command, Abraham sacrificed his comfortable life as he knew it to journey to a strange and foreign land (Gen. 12:1).

There are countless other stories of heroes who made incredible sacrifices such as Gideon (Judg. 6–8), Samson (Judg. 13:24–16:31), David (1 Sam. 16, 1 Kings 2), Daniel (Dan. 6), Paul (Acts 7:58–28:31), Samuel (1 Sam. 1–28), and all the prophets.

The fact is, success at anything will take sacrifice and hard work. It will require that you make up your mind that you want to change—no matter what. Yes, change is scary, and your body and mind will fight against change, but know that God understands your fears, your weaknesses, and your disappointments, and will never give you more than you can bear (1 Cor. 10:13).

Today's Health Challenge

Share what adjustments you are going to make to reach your goal.

Additional Study

1. Read some more of the Bible greats who pushed pass their comfort level like Noah (Genesis 6:1–11:32) and Abraham (Gen. 12:1). What can you learn from them that will help you on your journey?
2. Reflect on your past attempts at losing weight. Were you willing to make the necessary sacrifices?
3. What is the Holy Spirit telling you about sacrifice and why it's important to your journey?

Today's Confession

I am as bold as a lion. I can endure to the end because You are my strength and shield. I have the capacity for victorious living. I operate in excellence and purpose to complete every task that I set out to do. I can do all things through Christ who gives me strength.

Workspace/Reflections

Week 1 Exercise

Day 1 - Boot Camp - Bike Ride

Day 2 - walk (hospital route)

Day 3 - walk (school route)

Day 4 - walk (Sunset Park)

Day 7 - walk (45 min.)

Make exercise a priority. Walk or bike everyday.

No candy & sweets! Eat fruit for snacks.

Day 3

COUNT THE COST: THE CONSEQUENCES OF INACTION

Scripture Reflection

"If you keep quiet at a time like this, deliverance and relief for the Jews will arise from some other place, but you and your relatives will die."
(Esther 4:14 NLT)

"Those who think they have no time for bodily exercise will sooner or later have to find time for illness." ~ Edward Stanley

Yesterday we looked at some of the sacrifices and costs associated with reaching your weight release goals. But have you ever thought about the costs associated with not reaching your goal? What will happen if you don't stop your poor eating habits? Your lack of physical activity? If you don't stop consuming so much sugar, fat, and calories? What will it cost your family? What will be the cost to your self-esteem? Your relationships? Your joy?

It's difficult to take a long, hard look at all the costs of unfulfilled goals and desires. Sometimes the pain is so difficult to face that we would much rather hide our heads in the sand than face the truth about how much pain we're causing ourselves. However, until we confront the pain that we're causing ourselves and others we'll never be motivated enough to want to move past it.

In the book of Esther, we see a woman faced with a difficult decision. Although she was a queen and enjoyed the benefits of the king's power and wealth, her position came with a price. She could have lived a comfortable life in a palace with a king, but the costs meant jeopardizing the safety of the entire Jewish race. An entire race may not be dependent on your weight loss but, then again, the legacy of health that you leave for your family might be. Will you leave them a legacy of blessings or curses?

Today's Health Challenge

Throughout the day today, complete the statement below. Write out at least seven different answers. Try your best to record them as you think about them instead of trying to remember at the end of the day. Reflect on your feelings as your day progresses.

The cost if I don't release the weight is ...
unhappiness with the way I look
back pain increases
The cost if I don't release the weight is ...
not able to do things I like - biking, etc.
overall health issues - heart, etc.
The cost if I don't release the weight is ...
clothes don't fit - change in wardrobe
overall sense of failure

Additional Study

1. Meditate on the future impact of your health on your family, your future, your legacy.

"If you keep quiet at a time like this, deliverance and relief for the Jews will arise from some other place, but you and your relatives will die."
(Esther 4:14 NLT)

2. Reflect on the importance of you being in good health. Does it encourage you or overwhelm you? Ask God to help you see the importance of being in good health without feeling any guilt or shame about your past.

3. Pray that your family will live a legacy of good health. Pray that every curse of poor health will be broken.

Today's Confession

All things work together for good. My pain will turn into laughter, my cross will be exchanged for a crown, and my mourning will be turned into dancing. I am blessed and I am a blessing. My disappointments of the past will be turned into testimonies in the name of Jesus.

Workspace/Reflections

Day 4

UNDERSTANDING THE PROCESS: LITTLE BY LITTLE

Scripture Reflection

"Little by little I will drive them out before you until you have increased enough to take possession of the land." (Exodus 23:30 NIV)

"Take the first step in faith. You don't have to see the whole staircase, just take the first step."
~ Martin Luther King, Jr.

How many years did it take you to gain your excess weight? Even though it may have taken you many years to gain weight, we tend to want to lose weight quickly.

Programs like "The Biggest Loser" have created the illusion that weight loss is quick. They show people losing 25 pounds in a week. However, the fast track is never the right path. Change comes through renewing your mind daily with the Word of God. It's a process that happens day by day, little by little, step by step, from glory to glory. God's goal is Christ's fullness in our life. He wants to bring us to new levels and allow us to experience a life of freedom from all the things that keep us bound.

As the Israelites marched out of Egypt through the Red Sea and into the wilderness, God promised he would be with them through the entire journey. He also promised that he would help them have victory over all of their enemies and was very specific about how He would help them. God says, *"I will drive them out little by little until you have increased enough to take possession of the land"* (Exod. 23:30). Why would an all-powerful God take his time to act? God understands that to be victorious, certain skills must be developed; such as persistence, patience, strategy, and submission. These qualities aren't developed overnight. God wants us to get the lessons as well as the blessings. Success comes step by step.

Are you also prepared to take it step by step, little by little?

Today's Health Challenge

Adjusting for setbacks and unforeseen circumstances, how much longer will it take you to reach your goal than you originally projected?

Additional Study

1. Meditate on Exodus 23:20. *"I will drive them out little by little until you have increased enough to take possession of the land."* Why did God drive them out little by little? to teach the Israelites patience, persistence, to trust Him
2. What does God want to increase in your life little by little? Patience, discipline, submission, sacrifice? Journal your response.
3. Reflect on your past attempts at quick weight loss. What was the result?

Today's Confession

Thank You for Your promises. I am making progress. From victory to victory, success to success, I am getting stronger each day. I am more than an overcomer. I am advancing in everything I put my mind to. I am unstoppable!

Workspace/Reflections

2. Discipline

God is teaching me discipline when make choices of what I eat.

3. Lose the weight then go back to old habits.

Yesterday while walking it was the first day I felt more energized & not lethargic. When I got up in the night I felt good - not heavy & bloated. No tums at bedtime! I can feel the difference eating healthy makes.

Day 5
SUBMIT TO GOD

Scripture Reflection

"And the LORD went before them by day in a pillar of a cloud to lead them the way; and by night in a pillar of fire, to give them light; to go by day and night." (Exodus 13:21 KJV)

"You cannot fulfill God's purposes for your life while focusing on your own plans." ~ Rick Warren, The Purpose Driven Life

Just what does it mean to you to submit your weight loss program to God? Do you even know what it looks like? Being open to His leading and prompting? Admitting to Him your inability to do it without Him? Inviting Him to partner with you? Hearing only what He is telling you through your journal entries and prayer time? These are all practical forms of submission.

If we could lose weight (or rid ourselves of any other stumbling block) on our own, then we wouldn't need God. Strong willpower, self-discipline, and self-control may help you reach your goals, but chances are the journey won't be enjoyable and definitely isn't sustainable. Instead of always getting frustrated trying to do it your way and wasting time, money, and your health, the first and most important step is to submit your weight loss program to God.

God gives us a beautiful illustration of how He wants us to live with Him. From the time of the exodus until the Israelites entered the Promised Land, the Lord led them by day with a pillar of cloud, and by night with a pillar of fire. God is just as faithful to us if we allow Him to lead. Although it may not be by clouds and fire it may be that still small voice, the confirmation from a friend, or the inner feeling of peace. He also promises us that He will never leave us or forsake us.

You CAN rest from all of your efforts—no more crazy diets or gimmicks, no more wasted money, no more frustration, and no more guilt or condemnation. Starting today, refuse to take another step in your health program without God.

Today's Health Challenge

What conscious behaviors and actions are you currently engaging in that show your lack of submission in the area of your weight loss process. List 5-10 of them and then begin asking the Holy Spirit to help you. Say each one of them aloud.

Additional Study

1. Meditate on knowing that God's presence is with you day and night.

"And the LORD went before them by day in a pillar of a cloud to lead them the way; and by night in a pillar of fire, to give them light; to go by day and night."
(Exodus 13:21 KJV)

2. Reflect on His desire and promise to lead you and guide you. How does this help you to submit to Him?

> *"And the Lord will guide you continually and satisfy your desire in scorched places and make your bones strong; and you shall be like a watered garden, like a spring of water, whose waters do not fail."*
> (Isaiah 58:11)

3. Take time to rest in God's presence and ask Him to help you submit. Listen to His response to you and ask Him to reveal His presence to you so you can feel confident in His presence.

Today's Confession

I walk in Your presence today. I choose to honor You, God, by what I eat, and in all I do. I submit my weight, my health, and my body to You. I walk with courage, discipline, and perseverance in times of testing and temptation. I am blessed and prosperous in You.

Workspace/Reflections

Week 2 Exercise

Monday 9.26.22 141.5 -3 lbs. :)

Mon - boot camp

Tues - walk high school / hospital

Fri - walk @ What Cheer

Sat - bike ride 7 miles Belva Deer (hills)

Sun - walk high school

out of control eating & poor habits

Looking to food for comfort - bad day?

eat chocolate.

Tried to do it in my own strength &

will-power. Haven't prayed about it.

Doubts as to whether it will work

"this time"

Haven't included the Lord before in this journey.

Day 6
THE POWER OF PRAYER

Scripture Reflection

"Pray that you will not fall into temptation."
(Luke 22:40 NIV)

"Pray more, worry less."

Is it really necessary to bring prayer into your weight loss program? If you believe in the power of prayer then your answer should be a resounding, 'yes!' Yet far too many Christians have never thought of praying about their weight loss. Some people have the belief that praying for your weight loss is too petty a request to bring to God, especially if you feel like you brought it on yourself. But nothing could be further from the truth. If it pains you and is hindering you from living the life Christ died for you to have then it's important to God, too. There is no prayer too big or too small for God.

Hands down, prayer is the most effective and precious gift that God has given us. It is an intimate time of communication with God. He invites us to request what we need and then trust Him to meet our needs.

The power of prayer is life-changing. The more we reach out to God in prayer, the more we experience His transforming peace. Through prayer we war against our strongholds, we replace our fear with faith, and we receive His peace when nothing around us is peaceful. Through prayer, God's power gets downloaded into us.

Jesus asked the disciples to pray so that they would not fall into temptation (Luke 22:40). He knew that they were going to face many difficulties and wanted them to be proactive. After Jesus instructed them, He then walked away from them and prayed on His own. As He prayed, verse 43 says that *"an angel from heaven appeared and strengthened him"*.

Imagine praying and immediately being strengthened to continue your journey. The same God who strengthened Jesus in the garden is the same God who will strengthen you in all your journeys. Trust Him today to meet your needs by spending time in prayer with Him. God always delivers on His promises!

Today's Health Challenge

Prayer is one of our greatest weapons to war against the enemy, to align our will with God's, and to help us to resist temptations. Based on where you currently are in your walk, this may or may not be an overwhelming exercise for you. Your health challenge today is to boldly say your prayer out loud. You can do it in the mirror or wherever you feel comfortable.

Additional Study

1. Meditate on the importance of praying to God during temptations and trials

"Pray that you will not fall into temptation."
(Luke 22:40 NIV)

2. Ask the Lord to reveal Himself to you in prayer today.

   "But grow in the grace and knowledge of our Lord and Savior Jesus Christ. To him be the glory both now and to the day of eternity. Amen." (2 Peter 3:18)

3. Pray for your health today. As you pray, what is the Holy Spirit saying as you listen to His voice?

Today's Confession

I thank You that I don't have to be worried or anxious about anything. I bring my request to You with thanksgiving and stand with confidence that You will bring it to fruition. I know that You are able to do above all that I can ask or think.

Workspace/Reflections

Day 7
THE POWER OF CHOICE

Scripture Reflection

"Give yourselves completely to God, for you were dead, but now you have a new life."
(Romans 6:13 NLT)

"You are free to make whatever choice you want but you are not free from the consequences of the choice." ~ Unknown

In order for change to be permanent, God wants us to replace our old patterns and behaviors with new ways of thinking and behaving. These new behaviors must be continually applied until they are consistent and habitual in our lives. Otherwise, when we feel afraid and vulnerable we will revert to what we've always done.

Change will require the perfect blend of faith and action (James 2:26). Once you've submitted your weight release to God, He will prompt you to move to higher levels of success in this area and all other areas of your life. What is the Holy Spirit prompting you to change first? There are probably a whole lot of areas where you feel you need to change. Identify them and choose one that you are going to commit to changing immediately.

Get up! Go! Grow!

God called the Israelites to move from their present state of slavery to a life of freedom. Their journey was fraught with many challenges, and through them all the Israelites went back to what they knew best—grumbling, complaining, living in disobedience, and worshiping false idols.

The result? Forty years of wandering aimlessly for a journey that scholars estimate would take anywhere from 11 days to one year! Glory to God that He has given us a new heart and a new spirit that allows us to live by His rules and not our own (Ezek. 36:26-27).

Today's Health Challenge

Take some time and find a scripture you will recite to renew your mind every time you don't stick to your goal. As you make a daily choice to stay focused on your goal, God will honor your commitment and strengthen you on the journey.

Additional Study

1. How have you been choosing to stay in your current health situation instead of relying on God?
2. What choices could you make to show your trust in God and His best for you?
3. How will you walk in faith AND action?

"For as the body apart from the spirit is dead, so also faith apart from works is dead." (James 2:26)

Today's Confession

I am dead to sin. Your strength and grace has changed me and renewed me. I have a new life in You and do things that lead to holiness and joy. The power of Your life-giving Spirit has freed me from the power of sin. Your Spirit that controls my mind has given me life and peace.

Workspace/Reflections

Rom. 12:2

And do not be conformed to this world
(with its superficial values & customs)
but be transformed & progressively
changed (as you mature spiritually)
by the renewing of your mind
(focusing on godly values & ethical
attitudes) so that you may prove
(for yourselves) what the will of God is,
that which is good & acceptable &
perfect (in His plan & purpose for you)

He refreshes and restores my soul (life)
He leads me in the paths of
righteousness for His name's sake.
Ps. 23:3

Day 8

SPEAKING TO YOUR SITUATION: POWERFUL, POSITIVE AFFIRMATIONS

Scripture Reflection

"The tongue has the power of life and death."
(Proverbs 18:21 NIV)

"The greatest discovery of my generation is that human beings can alter their lives by altering their attitudes of mind." ~ William James

Affirmation is one of the most powerful tools God has given us to combat every single problem in our lives! The book of John starts off, "In the beginning was the Word ..." Huh? What does that mean? In Hebrew Scripture, the 'Word' was an agent of creation—so powerful that Psalm 33:6 states that, "The Lord merely spoke, and the heavens were created."

Is it possible that God has also given us this same power? Then God said, *"Let us make man in our image, to be like ourselves"* (Gen. 1:26). This includes the power to speak to our situations and circumstances. *"... you could say to this mountain, 'Move from here to there,' and it would move"* (Matt. 17:20).

Speak the Word of God over your life. When Jesus was being tempted in the desert, His greatest weapon was the Word of God. Three times Satan came at Him from different angles and all three times Jesus spoke the Word of God. He acknowledged that *"Man shall not live by bread alone, but by every word that proceeds out of the mouth of God"* (Matt. 4:4). What we say can give us life.

God gives us guidelines for how to powerfully use declarations. Always declare in the positive, "I am strong and courageous".

- Be clear and specific. (Jas. 1:6)
- Believe. (Matt. 17:20)
- Say them out aloud. (Ps. 119:13)
- Say them consistently; memorize them. (Ps. 119:9, 11)
- Don't beg or ask, but boldly declare. (Prov. 28:1)

Today's Health Challenge

In your journal, or using an electronic device, record how often you catch yourself saying something negative about yourself. Then write out a powerful affirmation today using the six points listed above. Memorize it and recite it throughout the day.

Additional Study

1. Meditate on the Scripture: *"The tongue has the power*

of life and death." (Proverbs 18:21 NIV) What does this scripture mean in relation to your health journey?

2. How is it that what you say reveals what's in your heart?
3. In what ways can you honor the Lord with what you say more often?

Today's Confession

I have the faith to move mountains. The Holy Spirit in me has made the impossible possible. I am more than a conqueror and I can overcome any obstacle that stands in my path. No weapon formed against me shall prosper. I am constantly making progress. I am a success.

Workspace/Reflections

Day 9
RAISE YOUR AWARENESS

Scripture Reflection

"Do not conform any longer to the pattern of this world, but be transformed by the renewing of your mind." (Romans 12:2 NIV)

"Let us not look back in anger, nor forward in fear, but around in awareness." ~ James Thurber

Do you often just go with the flow of life? Are you making things happen in life, or is life happening to you? If we are truly honest with ourselves, much of our life happens to us. We live on automatic pilot and accept the hand that life has dealt us. We are often not in control of the food choices we make. We grab something fast because we're in a rush. We eat because we have a craving for something, or someone gives us something to eat and we're too polite to say no.

This level of living keeps us stuck and robs us of our joy. Your successful weight loss will require you to tune in to all the choices you make, your thought patterns, your motivation for doing what you do, and even evaluate your decision-making process.

In the book of Daniel (1:8-14), Daniel, Hananiah, Mishael, and Azariah were faced with a dilemma where demands were placed on them. They were taken from their homeland and were told to eat food that wasn't part of their lifestyle or their custom. But Daniel and his friends resolved that they wouldn't eat the king's food. They had the Lord on their side, and if we allow Him into our lives so do we. Like Daniel, we must resolve to obey God rather than the pressures of this world. From Daniel we also learn that we must have a plan in place to resist temptation before it arises. He was determined to stay committed to his principles and choices.

In the New Testament book of Romans, we also learn the difference between living consciously by focusing our lives on Jesus versus living under the Law of Moses, which was ritualistic and only provided temporary relief. Romans 8:5 teaches us that, *"Those who are dominated by the sinful nature think about sinful things, but those who are controlled by the Holy Spirit think about things that please the Spirit."*

Today's Health Challenge

Today you will be 100 percent conscious of everything you put into your mouth. You will only eat foods that will build your body and not cause it any harm. This will take some additional planning on your part, so take some time before you leave the house to organize yourself. Avoid all processed foods, all fast foods, all additives and preservatives, and all sugar and caffeine.

Additional Study

1. Spend some time today reflecting on the importance

of being intentional about what you will and will not eat. How does that bring glory to God?

> *"But Daniel resolved not to defile himself with the royal food and wine, and he asked the chief official for permission not to defile himself this way."* (Daniel 1:8)

2. Meditate on why you want to live by the spirit. How does it keep you safe, protected, and out of harm's way?

> *"Those who are dominated by the sinful nature think about sinful things, but those who are controlled by the Holy Spirit think about things that please the Spirit."* (Romans 8:5)

3. Receive a fresh anointing of the Holy Spirit. Open your heart and become aware of His presence. Ask Him to make you more conscious and present to His presence. He is there to guide you and direct you if you let Him.

> *"Or do you not know that your body is a temple of the Holy Spirit within you, whom you have from God? You are not your own."* (1 Corinthians 6:19)

Today's Confession

I love You, Lord, and thank You for Your Spirit that lives in me. My mind is set on things above. I become more and more like You each day. I am created in Your image. I make responsible choices and decisions. I have the ability to solve my problems with You as my guide. I take authority over this day in the name of Jesus.

Workspace/Reflections week 3

10.3.22 142 lbs +.5

I'm discouraged. I feel like I am making good choices. I'm giving up desserts & candy. At restaurants I'm choosing to order salad. Yet no progress. But I feel better. I just came home from a camping weekend feeling good not bloated. I didn't over eat & I'm exercising. Gonna keep going!

Exercise

Mon - boot camp

Tues - walk (high school + 4 blks)

Wed - walk (short / rain)

Thurs - walk (high school / hospital)

Sat - bike 32 miles } Root River Trail

Sun - bike 18 miles

Day 10
WHAT'S STOPPING YOU?

Scripture Reflection

"I do not understand what I do. For what I want to do I do not do, but what I hate I do."
(Romans 7:15 NIV)

"Character is expressed through our behavior patterns or natural responses to things." ~ Joyce Meyer

Why is it that, in spite of our deep desire for weight loss, we continually make the same mistakes of poor food choices and other disempowering behaviors? Why do we continue to cling so tenaciously to patterns that don't serve us?

Truth is, most of our patterns are unconscious. We've held on to them for so long that we don't even realize that they keep us stuck. To finally be free of the things that hold us back, we must first identify our defeating patterns, behaviors, thoughts and choices, and turn them over to God. These 'dream-robbers' keep us from living the life we were born to live. Our assignment is to subdue and overcome these dream-robbers if we want to keep unwanted weight off forever.

Paul's struggle with sin was as real for him as it is for us. In Romans 7:15, we hear the cry of a desperate man so frustrated with his sin nature.

In Luke 5:8, Simon Peter also comes to grips with his sinful nature as he realizes that God is even interested in helping him catch fish! He remarks, "Depart from me; for I am a sinful man, O Lord."

Coming to grips with your sinful nature is the first step in allowing the Spirit of God to dwell richly in you; gradually replacing your fears and faults with Christ's freedom from what's been holding you back. Like Simon Peter and Paul, once we realize our sinful nature and understand how deeply it's ingrained in us then and only then can we begin to understand that Christ is the only one who can help us, if we're willing to allow Him.

Today's Health Challenge

Write one recurrent pattern or behavior that keeps you from reaching your goal. Now write how these behaviors have shown up in your life at the following stages. Until you completely surrender these behaviors over to God, they will continue to show up in your life.

Additional Study

1. Meditate on the power of God to change us from the inside out and bring our will under submission.

"What a wretched man I am! Who will rescue me from this body that is subject to death? Thanks be to

God, who delivers me through Jesus Christ our Lord!" (Romans 7:24-25)

2. Worship Jesus for the power that's available through Him to live not according to the flesh, but through His Spirit.

   "For God so loved the world that he gave his only Son, that whoever believes in him should not perish but have eternal life." (John 3:16)

3. How does coming to grips with your sin nature bring you freedom and peace?

   "Depart from me; for I am a sinful man, O Lord." (Luke 5:8)

Today's Confession

Have mercy on me, O Lord. You have searched me and helped me uncover my anxious thoughts. I now begin the process of rooting them out forever. I thank You for replacing my old behaviors with new ones that are pleasing to Your eyes. Because of Your love, I am dead to sin. I boldly take hold of Your power that gives me victory over sin.

Workspace/Reflections

craving for chocolate &. sweets.
Thinking I deserve a reward after
a hard day or when emotionally challenged.
Desire for something sweet after a meal.

Child:

Was I rewarded with candy?
Not that I remember

Teenager:

Adult:

Habit of eating chocolate after a meal
or when stressed.

Day 11
WHAT DO YOU BELIEVE?

Scripture Reflection

"They continued to follow their own gods according to the religious customs of the nations from which they came." (2 Kings 17:33 NLT)

"Growth demands a temporary surrender of security. It may mean giving up familiar but limiting patterns, safe but unrewarding work, values no longer believed in, and relationships that have lost their meaning." ~ John C. Maxwell

We all have things that we believe about ourselves. We may have been told them, or we may have internalized a belief as a result of something that's happened to us in our childhood. In relation to our health, some of these beliefs might sound something like this:

- God isn't concerned about the physical, it's what's inside that counts.
- Physical exercise profits little.
- Realistically, chances are I'll never be thin.
- I'll put all the weight back on again if I lose it anyway.

These beliefs or positions about life can sometimes get in the way of us reaching our goals. As we unconsciously carry these beliefs with us into adulthood, they often sabotage our plans and goals. These faulty beliefs impact our emotions, actions, and health. The breakthrough will require a change in these thought patterns.

In the book of 2 Kings, the Israelites begin their slippery slope into idolatry. Their desire was to serve God, but their actions led to idolatry and corruption. The king of Assyria saw firsthand how harshly God dealt with idolatry so he sent for priests to teach the Israelites how to worship the Lord. The problem was that the new settlers also continued to worship their own gods according to the religious customs of the nations from which they came. The result was their ruin.

Israel was conquered because it refused to focus on the one true God. They couldn't turn away from their old beliefs even though it led them away from God. What beliefs are you refusing to let go of? Understand the cost of holding on—it's not worth it.

Over the next few days, we will look at how our beliefs make us engage in unhealthy behaviors such as excuse-making, blaming, procrastinating, and emotional eating. We do them because they protect us from the pain of these deep-rooted beliefs. Noticing which ones you engage in is a big first step toward freedom.

Today's Health Challenge

For today's challenge, identify a limiting belief that sabotages your weight loss efforts.

Additional Study

1. Meditate on how following our culture instead of God can lead you away from God's best for you when it comes to taking care of your body.

   "They continued to follow their own gods according to the religious customs of the nations from which they came." (2 Kings 17:33 NLT)

2. Give all of your limiting beliefs to God and ask Him to help you change the way you see yourself, the world, and even Him. He is able.

3. Ask the Holy Spirit to lead you to a thought life that only believes God's truth. Decide today that you don't want to live apart from His truth and light.

Today's Confession

Your promises are for eternity. Every generational curse and everything spoke against my health are broken in the name of Jesus. I declare that I am in sound health in my body, mind, and spirit. I am strong and courageous and successful in everything I do. I meditate on Your Word day and night. He who the Son sets free is free indeed, and I declare my freedom in You.

Workspace/Reflections

Faulty beliefs:

I'll just gain the weight back

As you age you gain - its inevitable

I'm always going to have a "tummy"

Day 12
REASONS OR RESULTS: EXCUSE MAKING

Scripture Reflection

"I have no one to help me into the pool when the water is stirred. While I am trying to get in, someone else goes down ahead of me." (John 5:7 NIV)

"He that is good for making excuses is seldom good for anything else." ~ Benjamin Franklin

I can't lose weight because I don't have the time ... I can't afford it ... I can't afford a gym membership right now ... My kids need me. Do any of these sound familiar?

I took a course a few years ago where the facilitator made a powerful statement. He said, *"In life, there are reasons and esults—if you have a reason, then you didn't get the result."* So, which would you prefer—a good reason or a good result?

Excuse-making is one of the faulty patterns that keep us stuck. Excuses keep us from taking responsibility for our lives and our health. They rob us of our personal power and leave us feeling helpless to our circumstances.

Excuses in and of themselves are just the symptoms of an underlying problem. One of the most important steps in releasing excess weight is to uproot excuse-making and begin dealing with the real issues behind the excuses you make. It's impossible to change what you don't acknowledge.

There's a sad story in the book of John about a man who allowed his infirmity to become his way of life for 38 years! The story outlines a lame man waiting at a healing pool that was believed to heal whoever was the first person to step into the water after it was stirred by an angel of the Lord (John 5:1-9). Although he may have had a legitimate excuse (like most of us) for not going after what he wanted, he blamed his situation on other people not helping him. He complained that other people were always jumping ahead of him and that's why he couldn't receive his healing.

What reasons do you have for why you haven't received breakthrough in this area? As legitimate as our excuses may be God wants us to take 100 percent responsibility for our actions, and He has equipped us with the ability to do so.

Today's Health Challenge

Make a list of all the excuses (even the legitimate ones) you use to justify why you aren't at your ideal, healthy weight.

Additional Study

1. Jesus's response to the infirm man's excuses were simple, clear, and direct: *"Get up! Pick up your mat and walk."* (John 5:8) As you review your list of

excuses you wrote in today's health challenge, how is Jesus calling you to get up? Will you obey Him?

2. Reflect on the difference of feeling powerless and helpless versus feeling empowered by God's spirit living in you. How can you reject the feelings of hopelessness when it comes upon you?

"I have no one to help me into the pool when the water is stirred. While I am trying to get in, someone else goes down ahead of me." (John 5:7 NIV)

3. How can you move from excuses to action and rest in the truth of who God is in your life?

"Cast all your anxieties on him, because he cares for you." (1 Peter 5:7)

Today's Confession

Father, You've clothed me with strength and honor. You've empowered me to be strong and courageous. I reclaim my power in You by taking 100 percent responsibility for my thoughts and actions. I am blessed with the Holy Spirit to accomplish my weight loss goals. I will have a testimony in the name of Jesus.

Workspace/Reflections

I don't want to make exercise a "god".

I need time with Gary instead of going to the gym.

It's not polite to turn down a dessert that's offered to you.

I just don't have enough will power to
... not eat a 2nd helping
... give up that dessert / candy baked good

I'm getting older & weight gain is a part of life. (inevitable)

Re-think!

- Include God in my weight loss
- Balance time with family & exercise — walk / bike with Gary
- Pray when tempted by food instead of giving in
- Realize how much better I feel when I'm not eating junk & keep doing that!

Day 13
THE BLAME GAME

Scripture Reflection

"It was the woman who you gave me who gave me the fruit, and I ate it." (Genesis 3:12 NLT)

"I'm only going to stand before God and give an account for my life, not for somebody else's life. If I have a bad attitude, then I need to say there's no point in me blaming you for what's wrong in my life." ~ Joyce Meyer

A close friend to excuse-making is the blame game. In this game, you lose no matter how well you play. The blame game sounds something like this: "My husband/wife does the shopping so I have no control of what food is in the house". "It's my genetics." In this game, you are the poor victim and someone else is to blame for why you're overweight. Like excuse-making, ending the blame game will require you to take 100 percent responsibility for your actions.

The habit of blaming can be seen since the beginning of time. When God asked Adam if he ate the fruit, Adam blamed it on the woman. Then when God asked Eve if she ate the forbidden fruit, she blamed it on the serpent. As the story plays out, we also learn a universal principle that every action will always have a consequence.

As we see in the Garden of Eden, the moment we blame someone else for our actions we delay our success, because we waste time focusing on the wrong problem, we doubt our own abilities to reach our goals, and we divert our attention away from the real problem and deprive ourselves of the joy that God has for us. Follow God's plan for your life by refusing to blame anyone or anything for your lack of results.

Today's Health Challenge

Record the names of anyone you blame for participating directly or indirectly in your not having your ideal health and weight. Take responsibility by apologizing to them today and tell them that, effective immediately, you will take 100 percent responsibility for your health. If the person is deceased, you can still let God know that you forgive them.

Additional Study

Blaming began with the first sin ever committed in the Bible. It continues to cost us just as it did with Adam and Eve.

> *"And He said, ...'Have you eaten from the tree that I commanded you not to eat from?' The man said, 'The woman you put here with me—she gave me some fruit from the tree, and I ate it.' Then the Lord God said to the woman, 'What is this you have done?' The woman said, 'The serpent deceived me, and I ate.'"* (Genesis 3:11-13 NIV)

1. Why did Adam blame Eve, and why did Eve blame the serpent? Who was to blame?

2. What were the consequences of blaming, and what can you learn from them? (Genesis 3:27)

3. What scriptures minister to you when you feel like blaming others instead of taking responsibility?

Jeremiah 17:9
James 1:14

Today's Confession

Father, forgive me for usurping my responsibility to You for my health and wellness. Excellent health is mine; energy and vitality are mine. I am designed to reach higher levels of health from victory to victory, glory to glory, in the name of Jesus!

Workspace/Reflections

I have done this!

I blame genetics.

I've also blamed Gary. We both like sweets -

so temptation is always present.

Day 14
AVOIDING PROCRASTINATION

Scripture Reflection

"How long are you going to wait before taking possession of the remaining land the Lord, the God of your ancestors, has given to you?"
(Joshua 18:3 NLT)

"Procrastination may relieve short-term pressure. But it often impedes long-term progress."
~ John Maxwell

Procrastination is another serious barrier that stops us from reaching our goals. It's a lot more complex than just putting things off. Well-known psychologist Piers Steel published almost 800 studies on procrastination!

The root cause of procrastination stems from a problem with our relationship with ourselves, which directly implies a problem with our relationship with our Heavenly Father. Like many other strongholds, procrastination usually stems from some type of fear: fear of failure, fear of success, fear of being controlled, fear of intimacy, fear of separation, etc. The list can go on and on.

In the Old Testament, Joshua was chosen to be Moses' successor to lead the Israelites to the Promised Land. His greatest strength was his willingness to submit to God. As he assumed his new position, he couldn't help wondering why some of the tribes were procrastinating in possessing the land as God had instructed them. To combat this problem, Joshua took the initiative and delegated three men to take action and move the task forward.

This issue is far too complex to address in this book alone, but the Word offers some solutions to get you to start changing this destructive behavior of procrastinating.

A first step in overcoming procrastination is to submit all of your fears to God as you focus on the end result instead of the fear.

Today's Health Challenge

What is one main thing that you have been putting off in relation to your weight loss and why?

Feeling like I'm missing out by giving up eating sweets.

Additional Study

Fear of being left out – not belonging.

1. Which of the fears listed above could be contributing toward keeping you from taking action on your health and wellness goals?

2. Only five of the seven tribes received their inheritance. Why were they willing to settle for less than God's best? What kept them from receiving their inheritance? Can you identify similar patterns and

fear

behaviors in your life? Turn them over to God and ask Him to help you.

3. Joshua took charge of the situation and put a plan in place to advance the goal. How can you take charge of the main thing you've been putting off? What specific actions can you take to get started?

"Appoint three men from each tribe. I will send them out to make a survey of the land and to write a description of it, according to the inheritance of each. Then they will return to me." (Joshua 18:4)

Today's Confession

I seek Your kingdom above all else. I put You before my agendas, my timelines, and my priorities. I walk in faith and not fear. I walk in power, victory, and a sound mind. I do everything on time and in order. All my steps are ordered by You.

Workspace/Reflections

10.10.22 142 Week 4

I weighed in at 140.5 before we left for the weekend. Had a wonderful time in MN - rode 50 miles on Root River Trail but also ate wonderful food including some small portion desserts. Time to get back to work! Even though I ate what I wanted never felt stuffed. The exercise was great - pushed myself to accomplish big things.

Exercise

Mon - boot camp

Tues - walk long route

Sat - bike ride 13 miles

Sun - walk 2 miles

Day 15
OVERCOMING EMOTIONAL EATING

Scripture Reflection

"In your anger, do not sin: Do not let the sun go down while you are still angry, and do not give the devil a foothold." (Ephesians 4:26-27 NIV)

"Feel your feelings, don't feed them." ~ Unknown

Another destructive behavior that will always sabotage your weight loss program is emotional eating. Experts estimate that 75 percent of overeating is caused by emotions. Emotional eating is when we eat in response to our feelings, regardless of whether we're hungry or not, and/or when we use food as a tool or coping mechanism to either numb pain or to feel better. Common feelings that lead to emotional eating include boredom, stress (financial, relational, mental, etc.), loneliness, tiredness, and frustration.

In Ephesians 4, Paul teaches how to effectively deal with the stresses of life. He is talking more specifically about strife between people, but it also applies to dealing with our inner turmoil. He points out that it's okay to be angry (or experience other emotions), but we must find Godly ways of dealing with it. Unresolved issues give way to the devil operating in our lives.

The psalmist also tells us when we are angry to search our hearts and be silent (Psalms 4:4).

But the one thing that Jesus wants above all else is that you spend time listening to him, 'sitting at his feet', as it were. That needs to come first, before all these other things. That is where peace is found.

Over time you will learn how to develop appropriate and effective ways of dealing with your emotions such as:

- Taking the time to ask yourself what the underlying feeling is that's triggering the emotion.
- Submitting that feeling/situation to God; ask Him to handle it instead of food.
- Pausing. Emotional eating can be so intense, but if you can hold off for 10-15 minutes the craving will often subside.

Today's Health Challenge

What emotion led you to eat unnecessarily the last time? What was the underlying feeling?

Additional Study

1. Reflect on the scripture: *"Tremble and do not sin; when you are on your beds, search your hearts and be silent."* (Psalm 4:4) What does it mean to search your heart and be silent, and how can you apply that to your weight releasing journey?

Next time I'm frustrated & want to eat – stop &. pray.

2. Paul points out that it's okay to be angry (or experience other emotions) without acting out of them. What can you do instead, the next time you experience a strong emotion that's triggering you to eat? take a walk
3. Psalm 139:23 tells us to ask God to show us what's going on behind the surface of our emotions. Pray and ask God to show you what's at the root of your emotional eating.

"Search me, God, and know my heart; test me and know my anxious thoughts." (Psalm 139:23)

Today's Confession

He who the Son sets free is free indeed! I rejoice because I am free from bondage. I am free from emotional eating. I am free to be me, created in Your image and destined for greatness. I have the capacity to effectively deal with every situation and circumstance that my mind, people, or the enemy will throw my way.

Workspace/Reflections

Long car rides & in front of TV — eating out of boredom

Frustration at work or with others — crave chocolate

Day 16

ARE YOU A GIANT OR A GRASSHOPPER?: POOR SELF-IMAGE

Scripture Reflection

"We even saw giants there, the descendants of Anak. Next to them we felt like grasshoppers ...!"
(Numbers 13:33 NLT)

"See yourself as God sees you."

How do you see yourself when you look in the mirror? Do you focus on your strengths? Or, do your eyes home in on all the flaws? If we're honest with ourselves, most of us focus on all that's wrong with us rather than on what's right.

Poor self-image is one of the big dream-robbers. It can be the cause of procrastination, excuse-making, blaming, lack of faith, and lack of self-control—to name just a few. It will affect how you see the world and how you think the world views you.

In the story in Numbers, 10 men were sent to scout out land that God had promised the Israelites. The men returned with fearful stories of giants that would surely devour them, even though their reports conflicted with Joshua and Caleb's—two men with great vision and self-esteem. The 10 men had such low regard for themselves that they saw themselves as grasshoppers in comparison to their enemies. If you see yourself as small or incapable, or not worthy, then that's exactly what the world will reflect back to you.

Here's a biblical plan from this story to help you build your self-esteem:

- Believe what God says about you and what He has promised you regardless of what the majority of people (society, friends, and peers) might say about you.
- Have the right attitude. Caleb trusted God to give Israel the land He promised them.
- Stand firm and declare positive affirmations to combat negative ones. Caleb declared, *"We can certainly conquer it!"* (Num. 13:30)
- Learn to distinguish God's voice. God will never condemn you or make you feel bad.
- When the Holy Spirit convicts you of sin, he will always direct you toward a specific action that you can take (John 3:19-21).

Today's Health Challenge

Write down 10 things that you like about yourself.

Additional Study

1. Contrast Caleb and Joshua's report with the report

of the other scouts. Why did they see things so differently? What made the difference?

2. There's a stark contrast between how God sees us and how we see ourselves. Study one, two, or all of these scriptures to get a clearer picture of how God sees you so that you can start to realign your thinking.

I am far from oppression, and will not live in fear. (Isaiah 54:14)

I am loved lavishly by God. (1 John 3:1)

I am born of God, and the evil one does not touch me (1 John 5:18)

I am complete in Him Who is the head over all rule and authority—of every angelic and earthly power. (Colossians 2:10)

I am accepted in the beloved. (Ephesians 1:6)

I am alive with Christ. (Ephesians 2:5)

I have the mind of Christ. (1 Corinthians 2:16; Philippians 2:5)

I have the peace of God that surpasses all understanding. (Philippians 4:7)

The Spirit of God, who is greater than the enemy in the world, lives in me. (1 John 4:4)

I am renewed in the knowledge of God and no longer want to live in my old ways or nature before I accepted Christ. (Colossians 3:9-10)

I am born again—spiritually transformed, renewed and set apart for God's purpose—through the living and everlasting word of God. (1 Peter 1:23)

I am God's workmanship, created in Christ to do good works that He has prepared for me to do. (Ephesians 2:10)

I am a new creation in Christ. (2 Corinthians 5:17)

3. Give your feelings of low self-esteem and low self-worth over to God and ask Him to transform you into the likeness of Jesus today. Make space to let God fully love you, and ask the Holy Spirit to help you see yourself the way He sees you.

Today's Confession

I am fearfully and wonderfully made. I am the apple of Your eye. There is no condemnation for those who are in Christ Jesus. Through Christ Jesus, the Spirit set me free from the power of sin. I can certainly conquer this stronghold and any other one that will come my way, in Your matchless name!

Workspace/Reflections

hard-working

organized

motivated

think thru decisions

detail oriented

musical

loving/kind

truthful

Day 17
STAY SELF-CONTROLLED

Scripture Reflection

"Stay alert! Watch out for your great enemy, the devil. He prowls around like a roaring lion, looking for someone to devour." (1 Peter 5:8 NLT)

"I have learned that I really do have discipline, self-control, and patience. But they were given to me as a seed, and it's up to me to choose to develop them." ~ Joyce Meyer

On top of the unconscious patterns that can sabotage us, we also engage in many conscious patterns. Lack of control is the first of these behaviors that we will delve into.

We live in a world of extremes. Going without food or overeating both cause us to lose focus and control. Avoid the extremes in life. Popular 12-step programs caution against H.A.L.T. – don't allow yourself to get too hungry, angry, lonely, or tired. Extremes wear us out and inhibit our decision-making ability. Poor food choices are often made when we're so tired that our bodies crave an instant pick-me-up—which is usually unhealthy.

We learn from King David how the lack of self-control can lead us into deeper and deeper sin. 2 Samuel 11:1 opens with the subtle but powerful indictment of King David. It reads, *"In the spring of the year, when kings normally go out to war, David sent Joab and the Israelite army to fight the Ammonites."* Here we learn that, prior to falling into sin with Bathsheba, David chose to hang out idly at home with his thoughts instead of going to war with the other soldiers. We should ask ourselves the same question: "Are we operating in our purpose?" And if not, does that cause us to lose our focus and control?

Another example can be found in the New Testament. We learn what happens when we make ourselves too busy. We learn that Martha is gently corrected by Jesus for busying herself in the kitchen and stressing herself out, while Mary's choice to sit at Jesus' feet and listen to him teach is affirmed. (Luke 10:38-42):

> *"'Martha, Martha,' the Lord answered. 'You are worried and upset about many things...'"*
> (Luke 10:41)

God's solution for staying self-controlled is found in 1 Peter 5:9. It warns us to be attuned to when we may be vulnerable. It's during these times that the enemy will sweep in and take advantage of our weakened state and lead us astray.

Today's Health Challenge

Record times when you feel vulnerable and out of control. Under what circumstances do you experience this most often?

Additional Study

1. Both the story of David and Mary teach us valuable lessons about the dangers of not controlling ourselves. David was idle and Mary was too preoccupied. What can we learn from these two stories that can help us when we're vulnerable, too?
when we are idle get up & do something - go for a walk
2. How can you stay alert as 1 Peter 5:8 instructs?
3. What will be your strategy the next time you feel yourself losing control?
go for a walk
have a cup of tea
take a bubble bath

Today's Confession

I stand firm against the enemy and he flees. I keep my eyes fixed on You, God, because You are the author and perfecter of my faith. I stand firm in Your Word. It is my sword and my shield. Your Word is a light unto my feet and a light unto my path. It brings me comfort, protection, and strength in times of need.

Realize how important my quiet time is - make it top priority!

Workspace/Reflections

when tired - think I deserve a "food" reward.

Weekends & Camping Trips

Day 18
HOW TO STAY FOCUSED

Scripture Reflection

"'Why were you searching for me?'" he asked. "'Didn't you know I had to be in my Father's house?'" (Luke 2:49 NIV)

"When trouble comes, focus on God's ability to care for you." ~ Charles Stanley

It's so easy for us to get distracted, emotional, discouraged, or just plain tired. How do we maintain our focus when we don't feel like it? It's so easy to lose focus. We live in a society where we have so many demands placed on us that there's little time for rest or reflection, and since we're operating at full throttle we really don't know how to function when we don't have 10 things on our to-do list.

In the Bible, we see a sharp contrast between how Jesus stayed focused and how His disciples were constantly distracted. In the popular story of Peter's attempt to walk on water, we can learn a lot about focus. Peter started off well—he was actually doing it! Then Peter experienced the same issue many of us experience.

He took his eyes off his goal and focused on the overwhelming situation. The result? He sank. If we focus on the challenges and magnitude of weight release, then we'll also sink into despair. To stay focused on your weight loss goal when situations are difficult, focus on the power of the Holy Spirit rather than on your own weaknesses (2 Cor. 12:9).

- Jesus teaches us a lot about focus.
- Jesus often went away on his own to refocus and spend time with his Father. (Mark 1:35; Luke 5:16; Matt. 26:39). early in morning in seclusion
- Jesus used scripture to counter the attacks of Satan. (Matt. 4:1-11)
- Jesus resolved to stay the course regardless of the circumstances. (Luke 9:51)
- Jesus enlisted help and support of others. (Luke 10:1)

Today's Health Challenge

Write out the main things that cause you to lose focus of your weight loss goal.

Want pleasure now – dessert or chocolate – temptation

Additional Study

1. Reflect on the scriptures above to learn about Jesus' focus. What action steps can you incorporate from Jesus' life to keep you from getting distracted?
2. What scripture(s) can you meditate on to keep you from getting distracted?

3. Reflect on 2 Cor. 12:9 NIV. How can it minister to you when you're losing focus?

> *"But he said to me, 'My grace is sufficient for you, for my power is made perfect in weakness.' Therefore I will boast all the more gladly about my weaknesses, so that Christ's power may rest on me."*

Today's Confession

I have the mind of Christ. My mind is set on the Spirit, which is life and peace. My mind is being renewed day by day. The Holy Spirit lives in me and quickens me to do His will.

1. Quiet time priority
when tempted - pray!

2. Matt. 6:33
Phil. 4:8

10.17.22

Workspace/Reflections

Week 5 138.5 lbs -6 lbs. total

So excited to break the 140 barrier!

Mon - boot camp

Tues - walk

Wed - core & more + walk/run

Thurs - walk

Sat - walk

Sun - walk

Day 19

PARTNERSHIPS

Scripture Reflection

"He who walks with wise men will be wise, but the companion of fools will suffer harm."
(Proverbs 13:20 NASB)

"Accountability breeds response-ability."
~ Stephen Covey

Weight loss challenges tend to be a very isolating and lonely stronghold. No one wants their friends, family, and loved ones to know how much they're struggling, so people tend to isolate themselves and try to solve their problems on their own. Like many other strongholds, weight-releasing is not a journey that you should even attempt to do on your own.

As you go through challenges, you will need others around you who will motivate you, help build your integrity, and show you how loved and cherished you are. They can give you a different perspective than you may be able to see on your own and create a hedge of protection around you. Your partner will also give you the encouragement you need when you're unable to motivate yourself.

When you're down or frustrated, it's natural to call someone who will make you feel better. This person will usually offer you some encouragement and pump you up. This type of accountability is great, but it's not always the best thing for us. Sometimes we need counsel that will lovingly advise us that we're wrong, that we're being immature, or that we need to repent for our behaviors. In the Bible, Nathan was one such wise man. He knew that he had to confront David about his sin. He knew that the truth would hurt, so he had to come up with creative ways of showing him that he was wrong without getting David's back up (2 Sam.12). It took great courage and tact to speak to David in a way that would get him to see his mistakes. Your accountability partner should be able to speak to you in such a way.

Surround yourself with people who love you enough to correct you and want you to succeed. Begin to pray that God would show you who your accountability partner should be. Having an accountability partner will require a high level of transparency and honesty.

Be vulnerable, honest, and willing to hear what your accountability partner has to say. The truth sometimes hurts. No one likes facing their 'dark side' or feeling like their 'stuff' is being exposed, but trust that these steps are beneficial for your growth and eventual victory.

Today's Health Challenge

Write down all of the people who will be supporting you on this journey. Gary, mom, Cheryl

Additional Study

1. Proverbs 13:20 highlights one of the benefits of having accountability, i.e. wisdom. What are some other benefits for you? Keeps me from going off deep end
2. Nathan was able to 'lovingly' confront David about his sin. Is there someone in your life bold enough to confront you when you sin?
3. Pray for your accountability partner right now. If you don't have one, pray that God will show you who you can ask.

Today's Confession

I confess my sins to another as You have instructed. I thank You for my partner and I thank You that we're able to sharpen each other. As iron sharpens iron, we sharpen each other. We stand in agreement to manifest what You have already done in heaven right here on earth!

Workspace/Reflections

Week 6 10.24.22 140.5 ☹

Walked more than ever - made some good choices but probably overate Sat & Sun evenings

Mon - boot camp

Tues - walk (cold)

Wed - walk

Thurs - walk Lake Darling

Fri - bike Lake Darling 137

Sat - walk

Had a great camping weekend - ate too much Sat night & had sweets but didn't totally derail.

Back to 139 but ready to keep going & finish the course!

Goal 2 weeks (or 3)

4 lbs!

Day 20
MAKING YOU A PRIORITY

Scripture Reflection

"You expected much, but see, it turned out to be little ... Because of my house, which remains a ruin, while each of you is busy with his own house."
(Haggai 1:9 NIV)

"Well-ordered self-love is right and natural."
~ Thomas Aquinas

What do you think is the No. 1 reason people give for not exercising? If you said 'time', you're 100 percent correct. And it may also be your No. 1 reason for not exercising and taking care of yourself as you should. Upon closer inspection, you'll see that the problem isn't really an issue of time (or lack of it), but rather an issue of values—what's truly important to you? You see, we give our time and attention to what we deem important to us. We say we want to lose weight, but more often than not this goal gets bumped to the bottom of our 'to-do' list. So, the real question becomes, "How important is losing weight to you?" Even though most of us would say it's very important, we're so stuck in our current routine that it's impossible to see how we could possibly fit anything else into the day.

In his book, *The Purpose Driven Life*, best-selling author Rick Warren teaches us that we have just enough time to do what God's called you to do, and if you can't get it all done it means you're trying to do more than God intended. Are there things in your life that take up too much of your time and don't leave you time to do the things you really want? Then it's time to take stock of what you really want and begin to reshape your schedule to make it a priority. When God is first in your life, He will help you to order your priorities and help you see that you need to be healthy in body, soul, and spirit in order to fulfill His calling on your life.

In the book of Haggai, we learn an important lesson about prioritizing our time. God had given the Jews an assignment to finish the temple when they returned from captivity. Like most of us they got busy, forgot their priorities, and grew apathetic to things that were once important to them.

Through Haggai, God challenged them to action: "'*You expected much, but see, it turned out to be little. What you brought home, I blew away. Why?*'" *declares the Lord Almighty.* "'*Because of my house, which remains a ruin, while each of you is busy with your own house.*'" (Haggai 1:9) Has God been calling you to rebuild your temple?

Today's Health Challenge

Making yourself a priority will often mean resetting your priorities by saying no to many other things that are vying for your time. Your challenge today is to say 'no' to all requests (non-work related) that are presented to you. Say 'no' to all lunch offers, phone conversations, etc. Practice the art of saying 'no' all day long, and share your experience with your accountability partner.

Additional Study

1. Like Judah's, our problem is also with misguided priorities. Take some time and reflect on where God fits into your priorities. Is He first?

2. There are consequences to not giving God first place in your lives. In the book of Haggai, we learn that the Jews' work was not productive and they were unfulfilled with their material possessions. What are some of the consequences you're experiencing with not putting God first?

   "You have planted much, but harvested little. You eat, but never have enough. You drink, but never have your fill. You put on clothes, but are not warm. You earn wages, only to put them in a purse with holes in it." (Haggai 1:6)

3. How will making God a priority help you to make yourself more of a priority?

Today's Confession

Father, I thank You that when I put You first You teach me how to prioritize. My steps are ordered by You. I do first things first. I seek Your kingdom above all else, and in doing so You teach me how to make the most of my day. In all I do, I worship You. My time is in Your hands and You have blessed it and given me good success.

Workspace/Reflections

week 7

mon - boot camp 139

Tues - walk 30 min.

Wed - walk 45 min

Thurs - walk 45 min.

week 8

Mon - boot camp 138

tues / wed / Thurs / Sun walk

week 9 137.5

today was my goal date. I am 3 lbs. short of goal. 1½ weeks until Thanksgiving. I will keep walking! Trying to keep walking even when cold & dark.

Day 21
STAYING ON COURSE

Scripture Reflection

"Whether you turn to the right or to the left, your ears will hear a voice behind you, saying, 'This is the way; walk in it.'" (Isaiah 30:21 NIV)

"You are the only real obstacle in your path to a fulfilling life." ~ Les Brown

Do you know when you're on the right track? How do you know that this time it's going to work? Morning devotion time, maintaining a food journal, bringing your lunch to work, grocery shopping each week, taking the time to plan your day, and taking the time to exercise are actions that make us feel like we're on track. They motivate us to stay the course and energize us to persevere for another day. These markers, or guideposts, are effective tools that keep us on track. Once we follow the guidepost, we're guaranteed to get where we're going.

Don't be afraid to try something new—it might not work, but it's okay. Making a poor decision doesn't mean we're forever out of God's will. That's the beauty of Scripture. It contains story after story of people who made bad decisions, but God still used them mightily. Two examples include Abraham (Gen. 12:11-13) and David (2 Sam. 11). They both did things that were clearly wrong, but God worked through them to accomplish great achievements. God can use all of our decisions, whether they're right, wrong, or neutral. What's important is that you get on course and listen for God's voice to direct you.

God wants to show you the path that you should follow. He has given us the promise, "My sheep hear My voice." There are many examples of great men and women in the Bible who listened for God's voice and then acted as a result (Hab. 2:2; I Kings 19:12). Like Habakkuk, a good tool for communicating with God is to journal what He is saying to you. Try writing out a question to Him and wait for his response. You can 'test it' once He responds by searching the Scriptures for confirmation.

Today's Health Challenge

In this study, we identified many areas that might be preventing you from reaching your healthy weight. What are some of the areas the Holy Spirt has identified that have been keeping you from your health goals? Write them out in the workspace below.

Additional Study

1. When the Jewish people left God's path, He guided them back to the right path. Are you willing to hear and heed His voice of correction when He offers it? Meditate on Isaiah 30:21.
2. What are some of the guideposts that will keep you on track?

3. As you listen to God's voice, what are the next steps He's leading you toward in your health journey?

"Commit your actions to the LORD, and your plans will succeed." (Proverbs 16:3)

Today's Confession

Thank You that You've promised that You will never leave me or forsake me. You are my teacher and my guide. Your ways are always right and true. I hear Your voice in all I do. Your Word guides me in all I do. I fix my eyes upon You, and Your Spirit gives me direction.

Prov. 16:3

Commit your works to the Lord
(submit and trust them to Him)
And your plans will succeed
(if you respond to His will and guidance)

Workspace/Reflections

PUTTING IT ALL TOGETHER

I commend you and congratulate you for your courage and determination to be in the best health that will glorify your heavenly Father.

You have now laid the groundwork for a deeper and more intimate relationship with your body and with the Creator of your body.

Remember that this is just the beginning. There's still much work to do, and I encourage you to continue to reach for greater heights in the Lord and in your health. Each new level brings new goals, new blessings, and a deeper understanding of who you are in Christ.

He created you to be whole and complete. He wants you to lack nothing. He loves you unconditionally and wholeheartedly, and He wants you to love yourself the same way. It brings your Father glory when you take care of His temple—it's one of His gifts to you.

As a kingdom citizen, rest in the fact that all things have been placed under your feet. You have victory over your weight challenges and every other stronghold that attempts to defeat you. You have been given that authority, and now it's time use it.

To effectively exercise your authority, you'll have to study and pray God's Word until you're firmly rooted in Him. Develop the new discipline of speaking the Word of God over your weight, your health, and your entire life. It will dramatically change you. Use the additional scriptures included to continue to meditate on the Word of God.

I recommend that you review this book periodically to help ingrain the new habits and track your spiritual growth. Or do our Weight Loss, God's Way 21-Day Challenge online alone, with a friend or with a group. The challenge adds a daily video skit/insight from me, music videos and community to the lessons in this book. You can take the challenge anytime but we also host 'live' challenges three times a year, where hundreds of women go through it together with weekly video recap meetings.

21daysgodsway.com

It is my prayer that these biblical principles to weight loss will lead you to a long life of excellent health, peace, freedom, and joy.

THANK YOU

Thank you for being motivated, courageous, inquisitive and committed to go deeper in your health journey and uncover the missing piece- Christ!

I pray that these principles have been as much of a blessing to you as they have been for me and the hundreds of thousands of women around the world that have experienced what it means to include God in their health and weight-releasing journey.

If you've been blessed by this book, then please don't keep it a secret!

There are millions of women who need to hear this message. Please take a moment to leave an honest book review so more people can discover this book as well.

This book has laid out a great foundation for you, but there's so much more for you to discover. Please keep in touch with me so that you can stay in this conversation and continue to make your health a priority - God's Way. Plus I'll send you a free copy of my '3 Steps to Overcoming Emotional Eating' guide and a discount for an online version of this devotion, when you enroll for my weekly emails on successful weight loss, God's way.

weightlossgodswaybonus.com

Leader's Guide

Weight Loss God's Way 21-Day Challenge Leader's Guide

"Therefore go and make disciples of all nations, baptizing them in the name of the Father and of the Son and of the Holy Spirit, and teaching them to obey everything I have commanded you. And surely I am with you always, to the very end of the age."
Matt 19:20

Over the last two years we've been hearing from women all over the world that they used *Weight Loss God's Way* in their Bible Study group. Then we started getting phone calls from churches asking us if they could use our book for their Bible studies. It showed me the need to get this guide into the hands of leaders and ambassadors so they could help spread the message of faith and health.

If this book has truly changed your life and you want to pay it forward and bless someone else, prayerfully consider leading a group through the 21-Day Challenge in your community or church. Coming together as a group holds you accountable, and provides an opportunity to develop consistency within your faith. The best way to learn is to teach, so we believe that as you lead others you will also continue to grow in the Lord.

Healthy by Design ignites and mobilizes leaders who want to use their spiritual gifts and skills so that others can be transformed by the truth of God's Word.

Know that when you say 'yes' to minister to others, you are changing and affecting not only their lives but also the lives of everyone they come in contact with. You will find that as a leader you will feel more connected with the devotionals, as you will take on a sense of ownership and responsibility and will want to support your small group as much as possible.

This guide will give you the option of leading the 21-day challenge on-line (virtually) or in an in-person group (at your home, church or community center). As a leader, you must register your courses with us. Please register your group here:

https://www.cathymorenzie.com/become-a-bible-study-leader/

The 21-day challenge/devotional works best when participants work independently and follow up their independent study with leader-led, small-group interaction either in person or virtually. As the group leader, it's your responsibility to facilitate discussion and conversation and make sure that everyone gets the most out of the devotionals. You are not responsible for having all the answers to people's questions or re-teaching the content. That's what the devotional is for.

Your role is to guide the experience, encourage your group to go deeper into God's work, cultivate an atmosphere of learning and growth amongst a body of believers, and answer any questions that the group may have.

Ideas and tips to get the most out of the Small Groups Sessions

Whether you're leading an in-person group or virtually, you will set the tone for group. Here are some suggestions to help you run a successful group.

1. **Emphasize that it's about God.** Although we use biblical and practical principles to guide us on how to address strongholds in our lives, remember that it's always about God. Your role as a leader is to always point everyone to the cross. Be intentional about making this journey all about God.

2. **Partner up.** Have your group choose an accountability partner to go through the devotional with. It's always more encouraging when you can connect with someone on a regular basis, in addition to when you meet as a group.

3. **Keep a journal.** Encourage your group to use a supplemental journal. They can choose from an on-line journal like Penzu (penzu.com) or use an old school pen and paper. Either way, taking time to record your thoughts, feelings, inspirations, and directives from the Holy Spirit is a great way to maximize the experience.

4. **Be consistent.** Meet at the same time and location each week. This will help the group to organize their time and their schedules. Try to select a time that works best for everyone.

5. **Plan ahead.** Take time prior to the weekly study to think about how you will present the material. Think about a particular story or example that would add to the material. Think about the most effective way to make use of the time.

6. **Keep it intimate.** Keep the small group small. I suggest a maximum of 12-15 for in-person studies. This will create a more relaxed and transparent atmosphere so that people will feel safe to speak.

7. **Be transparent.** You can set the tone for the group by sharing your story. This will help people to feel safe and establish trust with them. When you speak, give personal examples from your own life and avoid phrases like 'some people' and 'Christians'.

8. **Be professional.** Always start and end the sessions on time. Communicate clearly if you see that you will be going over time. Apologize and let them know how much you respect their time.

9. **Bring lots of energy.** Let your passion for studying God's Word be evident. Remember that your energy level will set the tone for the entire group, so bring it!

10. **Pray.** It might sound obvious, but make sure that prayer is an intricate part of the entire process. Pray at the beginning and end of every session. Feel free to call on others to lead the prayers. During the session, you can have one person pray for the entire group. Have one person open and another close (ask for requests or select someone). You can also encourage the group to pray for one another. Lastly, don't forget to pray during the time leading up to the session.

11. **Keep it simple.** If the sessions get too complicated, people will find reasons not to attend. If you plan to serve snacks, keep it simple and nutritious. Don't plan weekly pot-lucks that will require the group members to do too much work.

12. **Be creative.** Feel free to add music, props, or anything that you feel will add to the environment and facilitate learning.

13. **Be comfortable.** Make sure there's adequate comfortable seating for everyone. Check the temperature in the room. Alert everyone to where the powder rooms are located.

Preliminary Preparation for Leading Virtual/ Online Studies.

- Be sure you have registered your session with us. If you haven't already done so, go to:

  https://www.cathymorenzie.com/become-a-bible-study-leader/.

- Pray and seek the Holy Spirit to receive confirmation that you should be leading this devotional.
- Get familiar with any social media tools that you will be using to communicate with participants. Suggestions include Facebook Live or Zoom.
- Determine the dates and times you'll be meeting with the group. Book four to five sessions in total: one preliminary session followed by three additional sessions. You can also add a follow-up session to see how participants are doing post-challenge.
- Begin to promote the event online. We will provide you with all of the promotional materials.
- Prior to the first meeting, make sure everyone purchases a copy of this book. Include a link where they can purchase it.
- Be sure to test your equipment, paying attention to sound quality and your internet connection.

- Say hello to commenters by name and respond to their comments.
- Talk freely and naturally. Don't attempt to script what you want to say.
- Ask a lot of questions and wait for a response. With Facebook Live, there is a delay of a few seconds.

Preliminary Preparation for Leading In-Home Studies.

- Pray and seek the Holy Spirit to receive confirmation that you should be leading this devotional.
- Determine with your group how long you want to meet each week so you can plan your time accordingly. Most groups like to meet from one to two hours, so adjust the format based on your time-lines.
- Promote the bible study through community announcements, social media, in your church bulletin, or simply call a few of your friends.
- Send out an email, create an event on Facebook, or send a message on social media announcing the upcoming study.
- Prior to the first meeting, make sure everyone purchases a copy of this book. Include a link where they can purchase it.
- Complete a weekly attendance form.

Suggested Group Plan

The suggested plan is for a four-week session. Here's a breakdown of the four weeks.

A Four-Week Session Plan

Session 1:

This session is designed to set the tone for the program and to make sure everyone is prepared for the journey. Review the orientation video.

A. Welcome everyone to the session and open the session with prayer.

B. Share a bit about yourself and go around the room and have everyone introduce themselves. Have each person share what their biggest challenge has been in losing weight. What are the challenges and stresses that they face? For virtual groups, have guests type in their comments.

C. Give an overview of the 21-day devotional and a brief overview of the Healthy By Design Program and the Weight Loss God's Way Core Programs. Explain that the 21-Day Challenge is the beginning of an ongoing process and more advanced programs are available on cathymorenzie.com or in our membership group christianweightlossgodsway.com, should they choose to continue.

D. Housekeeping Items:

- Explain format for the sessions.
- Confirm dates and times.
- Where powder rooms are.
- 'Rules' for sharing - no talking about trigger foods such as chocolate, cake, cookies, chips, etc.
- Commitment to confidentiality.
- Attendance each week (in-person groups).
- Snacks for in-person groups (have volunteers).

E. Stress the importance of trust and transparency.

F. Instruct the group to complete the next seven days before the next session. Encourage them to carve out some time each day to participate in the Facebook group and to complete the devotional. Find out what the best time is for them to complete the lessons

G. Ask group if they had questions about the orientation video.

H. Highlight some of the points covered in the orientation video.

Discuss the three habits to practice and have everyone share which of the three habits they're practicing. Encourage the group not to try to choose all three. Explain them in more detail if necessary.

Session 2:

This session is designed to recap the first seven lessons in the program, to keep the group engaged and to foster a sense of community.

1. Welcome the group.
2. Start with an opening prayer.
3. Ask the group what insights/breakthroughs/testimonials they encountered as a result of what the Holy Spirt has been showing them over the past week.
4. Acknowledge that some may have broken their boundaries. Say something like, "Don't beat up on yourself. Renew your mind and keep on going. You don't need to start over."

Highlight the first seven days of the challenge. Use the 'Conversation Starters' to trigger discussion or conversation. You don't need to cover all of these points. Select one or two points that are relevant to your group. Feel free to use them when needed and share them in your own voice.

Share your responses when appropriate.

5. At the end of the session, ask if there are any questions. Close the session in prayer.

Conversation Starters for Days 1-7

Day 1 - What is your goal?

- Ask a few members what their goals are.
- Commend group on taking bold step of starting. Make a big deal out of it.
- Remind them to only choose one goal. Feel free to adjust the goal whenever necessary.
- If their goal is to track their food, suggest tools such as www.myfitnesspal.com or 'loseit'.
- For those choosing not to eat after 7:00 pm, encourage them to pray about what they'll do when the urge to eat hits them (offer suggestions if you have any).
- For those choosing to exercise each day for 15 minutes, suggest they choose to exercise at the same time every day.

Day 2 - Count the cost

- Ask a few members what the costs are for them.
- Conversation starter: "One of the biggest reasons we don't change is because we're not willing to truly sacrifice. Stepping out of your comfort zone is difficult, especially when past experience may have taught you that it's not safe to do so. Be willing to get uncomfortable practicing the new habits, and refuse to quit before they become ingrained in your lifestyle."

- Stress the importance of planning for success.
- Encourage grace and patience. For example, if you ate at 7:05 instead of 7:00, don't beat up on yourself. It's probably a lot better than you were doing before.
- Realize that making one adjustment will shift a variety of other things in your life. If you go to bed earlier let your friends and family know, otherwise they'll still be calling you and demanding your time.
- Encourage the group to be specific when sharing the changes they'll make. For example, instead of saying you're going to wake up early, share a specific time you're going to wake up. Instead of saying 'make time to exercise', share specifically what type of exercise you plan to do. Instead of saying you're going to take time to plan your meals, share what your specific planning day will be. Instead of saying 'go to bed earlier', share what your new bedtime will be.

Day 3 - Consequences of Inaction

- Ask some of members what the consequences are for them.
- Conversation Starter: "The costs are too dear to not take action each and every day. Yes, sacrifice will feel hard. Yes, your flesh will cry out. Yes, it's easier to do nothing. Yes, you will feel like quitting, but I pray with you to stay the course regardless of how hard it gets.

Suffer the temporary pain of success now, rather than the permanent pain of regret. At the end of each day and at the end of our life, we want to hear our Heavenly Father say to us, "Well done, good and faithful servant." (Matt. 25:23)

Day 4 - Understanding the Process

- Ask if they've made adjustments to their original goal.
- Acknowledge how sobering it must be for some people to see how long it might take and how some might be excited.
- Whatever their feelings are, remind them that the battle is the Lord's!
- Remind them that it's about progress, not perfection.

Day 5 - Submit to God

- Ask the group what they need to submit to God.
- Clarify what submission means. When you talk about what you're submitting, recognize that we can't submit sugar or eating. It's what's behind why you eat sugar that you need to submit—it's the unmet core need. For example, you submit your need for comfort, your need to feel better, or your insatiable need for something fulfilling. Trying to submit the food to God leads to more failure, as you may still wake up tomorrow with the sweet tooth because you have not allowed God to fill that underlying need. Also, stress that it's not the food that's the problem, but rather the void (unmet core need) that the food is trying to fill.

- **Stress: God can only cover what you're willing to uncover.**

Day 6 - The Power of Prayer

- Have the group share prayers.
- Remind them that God wants to be involved in this area of your life, so call out to Him and He will faithfully help you in your times of need.
- Encourage them to memorize today's prayer or scripture and use it as often as they need it.

Day 7 - The Power of Choice

- Conversation Starter: Remember, we can't always choose our circumstances, but we *can* choose how we respond to them.
- Continue to use your prayer to guide you into making the right choices. Let your prayers dictate your thoughts, words, and actions.

Session 3:

The purpose of this session is to recap lessons 8-14 and to encourage the group to keep on going.

1. Welcome the group.
2. Start with an opening prayer.

3. Ask the group what insights/breakthroughs/testimonials they encountered as a result of what the Holy Spirt has been showing them over the past week.

4. Acknowledge that some may have broken their boundaries. Don't beat up on yourself. Renew your mind and keep on going. You don't need to start over.

5. Highlight each of the lessons by using some of the conversation starters below.

6. End with a closing prayer.

Conversation Starters

Day 8 - Speak to Your Situation

- Ask the group if they are conscious of how they speak to themselves. Is it positive or negative?

- **Conversation Starter:** Stress how important words are. Your thoughts become your words, your words become your actions, your actions become your habits, and your habits shape your life. Try to stay present to what you say about yourself each day. Remember that words have power, so speak life and not death over yourself.

Day 9 - Raise Your Awareness

- **Conversation Starter:** Stress the importance of thinking about what we're thinking about all day long. God is here with you right now and He wants to make His presence known. Maybe you can't feel Him, but He's here. Loving you, encouraging you, and affirming you. He's not in the past, looking back at your mistakes, or in the future, pressuring you to do better. He is here, right now, right where you are.

Day 10 - What's Stopping You?

- Congratulate the group on making it to the (almost) halfway point.
- Acknowledge that we're going deeper and things might get 'tougher'.
- Acknowledge their courage to go deeper.
- **Conversation Starter:** I commend you all on having the courage to search the deeper parts of you that you may have consciously or unconsciously buried. It doesn't always feel good to open old wounds but it's necessary because our band-aid solutions aren't working. We need God's total, complete, and permanent healing. Let's continue to pray for and encourage each other!

Day 11 - What Do You Believe?

- Be empathetic to the brokenness and hurts that have been shared.
- Ask group to share some limiting beliefs that have impacted their health.
- **Conversation Starter:** Our flesh may want to quit now because it doesn't want to relive the pain that we experienced as children, but hold firm to the belief

that the Lord will cover what we're willing to uncover. So continue to be transparent and trust that God will cover you and mend all the tattered and frayed pieces in your life. Stay put and endure this journey to the end and receive your blessing. This is a sacred space and God is moving in the midst of your lives to restore the breech.

Day 12 - Excuse Making

- Congratulate and acknowledge their courage to share the painful issues.
- Ask the group what some of their excuses are for not taking action towards their health.
- **Conversation Starter:** As we unpack a lot of heavy and painful issues, give yourself a lot of grace and love. Refuse to wear any guilt, shame, or condemnation— it's not your fault. Believe that your future is bright as you walk this journey, with Christ undergirding your every step. Many of the things that happened to you in your past are not your fault. But now, as adults, it's your responsibility to change it.
- Ask if anyone will take on the exercise of contacting the person they've been blaming and apologize to them, or write a letter if the person is no longer alive.

Day 13 - The Blame Game

- **Conversation Starter:** Many of us have very legitimate causes for why we developed poor eating habits or why we're inactive. Many of us experienced abuse, abandonment, neglect, and shame at the hands of those who were supposed to care for us, and so we feel quite justified to cast blame.

Except we're all grown up, and as adults we now have a responsibility to right the wrongs that were done to us. Spending the rest of our lives blaming them will only keep us from receiving the love and peace that God has for us.

When we choose to take responsibility for all of our actions, we will experience a satisfaction unknown to those who blame and make excuses.

Day 14 - Overcoming Procrastination

- **Conversation Starter:** Believe it or not, our procrastination is directly related to our level of trust in God. If we really trusted Him at His word then we wouldn't hesitate. If we really believed what His Word says, then we wouldn't worry about failing, losing control, getting overwhelmed, being judged, or any of the other fears that keep us procrastinating. I pray that you will take time and discover how trustworthy our Heavenly Father is.

Session 4:

The purpose of this session is to recap days 15-21 and to encourage the group to continue to step 2.

Think about how you'll make the final session memorable. Maybe end with a nutritious meal, exchange written gifts, or organize something small that symbolizes God's love.

1. Welcome the group.
2. Start with an opening prayer.
3. Ask the group what insights/breakthroughs/testimonials they encountered as a result of what the Holy Spirt has been showing them.

Suggested Discussion Starters For Days 15-21

Day 15 - Overcoming Emotional Eating

- Ask group how pervasive emotional eating is in their lives.
- Find out what emotions trigger their emotional eating.
- Mention the breakthrough course in step 2 which focuses on getting to the root of emotional eating.
- **Conversation Starter:** Purpose to spend more time with God, and our feelings will be transformed into convictions and Godly wisdom about our health and all other areas of our lives.

Many of our emotions can only be met through fellowship with our Heavenly Father. Though our emotions may rage out of control, peace is a gift that can only be found when we seek the heart of God.

Day 16 - Self-Image

- Ask the group how difficult or easy it was for them to do the exercise.
- **Conversation Starter:** God longs for us to love Him and be loved by Him. When we can understand this our self-confidence will be through the roof! Our self-esteem comes from knowing that we are loved lavishly by God and He created us in His image. Let that be our main reason to hold ourselves in high esteem!

Day 17 - Self-Control

- Ask the group what causes them to feel out of control.
- **Conversation Starter:** When we acknowledge our weakness we gain the help of an Almighty, all-loving, ever-present God. Let's stop looking for willpower in ourselves and look to God as our strength. The real secret to self-control is God-control!

Day 18 - Stay Focused

- Ask the group what causes them to lose focus.
- Encourage the group to stop obsessing about the number on the scale and all the parts of themselves that they need to 'fix'.
- **Conversation Starter:** When you choose to focus your life on Christ, He'll do magnificent things in you

today. Follow the path of focus Jesus laid out for us as we choose to be about our Father's business.

Day 19 - Accountability

- Ask them who their accountability partner is.
- **Conversation Starter:** Accountability calls you to a higher standard when you don't feel like being your best. It increases your prayer power and gives you a safe space to be transparent and vulnerable, yet it doesn't let you off the hook when you're slipping. God has called us to be in relationship with Him and others so don't feel like you have to do thing on your own.

Day 20 - Making You a Priority

- Ask, "What do you need to say 'no' to in order to say 'yes' to yourself?"
- **Conversation Starter:** For many of us Christian women, the idea of putting yourself first may sound selfish and contrary to what we've been taught, but think about it... How can you take care of anyone else if you don't have the physical, spiritual, mental, and emotional health and strength for yourself? You're so worth it!

Day 21 - Putting it All Together

- Ask what was most impactful about the program.

- Ask for testimonials!

Congratulate group on completing the challenge.

Remind them that change isn't a one-time program. It's an ongoing process of continually submitting our needs and desires to God. God is continually transforming us day by day, from glory to glory.

Share about the Breakthrough program.

- Gain powerful insights and tools to help you get to the root of your weight issues.
- Gain understanding of your recurring cycle of unconscious behaviors and develop a strategic plan to overcome them.
- Explain that members can go to www.christian-weightlossgodsway.com to register. Wrap up session with closing words/thoughts.

End session with a closing prayer.

Thank you again for taking the time to lead your group. You are making a difference in the lives of others and having an impact on the kingdom of God.

Appendix

Additional Scriptures

Day 1 – GOAL-SETTING

Philippians 3:13-14 – *Brothers, I do not consider that I have made it my own. But one thing I do: forgetting what lies behind and straining forward to what lies ahead, I press on toward the goal for the prize of the upward call of God in Christ Jesus.*

2 Chronicles 15:7 – *But you, take courage! Do not let your hands be weak, for your work shall be rewarded.*

2 Peter 3:18 – *But grow in the grace and knowledge of our Lord and Savior Jesus Christ. To him be the glory both now and to the day of eternity. Amen.*

Philippians 4:12 – *I know how to be brought low, and I know how to abound. In any and every circumstance, I have learned the secret of facing plenty and hunger, abundance and need.*

Day 2 – COUNT THE COSTS

Hebrews 5:8 – *Although he was a son, he learned obedience through what he suffered.*

Romans 12:1 – *I appeal to you therefore, brothers, by the mercies of God, to present your bodies as a living sacrifice, holy and acceptable to God, which is your spiritual worship.*

2 Corinthians 6:14 – *Do not be unequally yoked with unbelievers. For what partnership has righteousness with lawlessness? Or what fellowship has light with darkness?*

Acts 17:26 – *And he made from one man every nation of mankind to live on all the face of the earth, having determined allotted periods and the boundaries of their dwelling place ...*

Day 3 – CONSEQUENCES OF INACTION

Proverbs 14:12 – *There is a way that seems right to a man, but its end is the way to death.*

James 4:17 – *So whoever knows the right thing to do and fails to do it, for him it is sin.*

James 4:3 – *You ask and do not receive, because you ask wrongly, to spend it on your passions.*

Day 4 – UNDERSTANDING THE PROCESS

Proverbs 13:11 – *Wealth gained hastily will dwindle, but whoever gathers little by little will increase it.*

Luke 16:10 – *One who is faithful in a very little is also faithful in much, and one who is dishonest in a very little is also dishonest in much.*

Proverbs 24:27 – *Prepare your work outside; get everything ready for yourself in the field, and after that build your house.*

Day 5 – SUBMISSION

2 Corinthians 5:17 – *Therefore, if anyone is in Christ, he is a new creation. The old has passed away; behold, the new has come.*

John 14:26 – *But the Helper, the Holy Spirit, whom the Father will send in my name, he will teach you all things and bring to your remembrance all that I have said to you.*

Proverbs 3:6 – *In all your ways acknowledge Him and he will make your paths straight.*

Day 6 – POWER OF PRAYER

John 14:14 – *If you ask me anything in my name, I will do it.*

1 John 5:14-15 – *And this is the confidence that we have toward him, that if we ask anything according to his will he hears us. And if we know that he hears us in whatever we ask, we know that we have the requests that we have asked of him.*

James 5:18 – *Then he prayed again, and heaven gave rain, and the earth bore its fruit.*

Day 7 – MAKING POWERFUL CHOICES

Proverbs 14:12 – *There is a way that seems right to a man, but its end is the way to death.*

Matthew 7:13-14 – *Enter by the narrow gate. For the gate is wide and the way is easy that leads to destruction, and those who enter by it are many. For the gate is narrow and the way is hard that leads to life, and those who find it are few.*

Exodus 21:24-25 – *Eye for eye, tooth for tooth, hand for hand, foot for foot, burn for burn, wound for wound, stripe for stripe.*

Day 8 – POWERFUL AFFIRMATIONS

Psalm 119:13 – *With my lips I recount all the laws that come from your mouth.*

Psalm 40:9 – *I proclaim righteousness in the great assembly; I do not seal my lips, as you know, O LORD.*

Psalm 22:22 – *I will declare your name to my brothers; in the congregation I will praise you.*

Day 9 – RAISING YOUR AWARENESS

Romans 12:2 – *Do not be conformed to this world, but be transformed by the renewal of your mind, that by testing you may discern what is the will of God, what is good and acceptable and perfect.*

2 Corinthians 4:16 – *So we do not lose heart. Though our outer self is wasting away, our inner self is being renewed day by day.*

Day 10 – COMING TO GRIPS WITH OUR SIN NATURE

1 Peter 5:8 – *Be sober-minded; be watchful. Your adversary the devil prowls around like a roaring lion, seeking someone to devour.*

1 John 3:8 – *Whoever makes a practice of sinning is of the devil, for the devil has been sinning from the beginning. The reason the Son of God appeared was to destroy the works of the devil.*

1 Corinthians 10:13 – *No temptation has overtaken you that is not common to man. God is faithful, and he will not let you be tempted beyond your ability, but with the temptation he will also provide the way of escape, that you may be able to endure it.*

Romans 12:2 – *Do not be conformed to this world, but be transformed by the renewal of your mind, that by testing you may discern what is the will of God, what is good and acceptable and perfect.*

Day 11 – WHAT DO YOU BELIEVE?

1 John 4:1 – *Beloved, do not believe every spirit, but test the spirits to see whether they are from God, for many false prophets have gone out into the world.*

Philippians 3:13 – *Brothers, I do not consider that I have made it my own. But one thing I do: forgetting what lies behind and straining forward to what lies ahead ...*

Romans 8:28 – *And we know that for those who love God all things work together for good, for those who are called according to his purpose.*

Day 12 and 13 – TAKING RESPONSIBILITY

Matthew 27:24 – *When Pilate saw that he was getting nowhere, but that instead an uproar was starting, he took water and washed his hands in front of the crowd. "I am innocent of this man's blood," he said. "It is your responsibility!"*

Genesis 43:9 – *I myself will guarantee his safety; you can hold me personally responsible for him. If I do not bring him back to you and set him here before you, I will bear the blame before you all my life.*

2 Samuel 14:9 – *But the woman from Tekoa said to him, "My lord the king, let the blame rest on me and on my father's family, and let the king and his throne be without guilt."*

Day 14 – AVOIDING PROCRASTINATION

Psalm 34:4 – *I sought the LORD, and he answered me; he delivered me from all my fears.*

Joshua 18:3 – *So Joshua said to the Israelites, "How long will you wait before you begin to take possession of the land that the Lord, the God of your fathers, has given you?"*

2 Timothy 1:7 – *For God did not give us a spirit of timidity but a spirit of power, of love and of self-discipline.*

Day 15 – OVERCOMING EMOTIONAL EATING

Ephesians 6:12 – *For we do not wrestle against flesh and blood but against the rulers, against the authorities, against the cosmic powers over this present darkness, against the spiritual forces of evil in the heavenly places.*

Ephesians 4:26 – *Be angry and do not sin; do not let the sun go down on your anger.*

Day 16 – SELF-IMAGE

Psalm 139:13-14 – *For you formed my inward parts; you knitted me together in my mother's womb. I praise you, for I am fearfully and wonderfully made.*

Genesis 1:27 – *So God created man in his own image, in the image of God he created him; male and female he created them.*

Ecclesiastes 3:11 – *He has made everything beautiful in its time. Also, he has put eternity into man's heart, yet so that he cannot find out what God has done from the beginning to the end.*

Ephesians 2:10 – *For we are his workmanship, created in Christ Jesus for good works, which God prepared beforehand, that we should walk in them.*

Genesis 1:31 – *And God saw everything that he had made, and behold, it was very good. And there was evening and there was morning, the sixth day.*

Day 17 – SELF-CONTROL

John 16:33 – *I have told you these things, so that in me you may have peace. In this world you will have trouble. But take heart! I have overcome the world.*

James 4:7 – *Submit yourselves, then, to God. Resist the devil, and he will flee from you.*

1 Peter 4:7 – *The end of all things is at hand; therefore, be self-controlled and sober-minded for the sake of your prayers.*

1 Corinthians 10:13 – *No temptation has overtaken you that is not common to man. God is faithful, and he will not let you be tempted beyond your ability, but with the temptation he will also provide the way of escape, that you may be able to endure it.*

Day 18 – STAYING FOCUSED

Psalm 119:15 – *I will meditate on your precepts and fix my eyes on your ways.*

1 Corinthians 7:35 – *I say this for your own benefit, not to lay any restraint upon you, but to promote good order and to secure your undivided devotion to the Lord.*

Philippians 4:8 – *Finally, brothers, whatever is true, whatever is honorable, whatever is just, whatever is pure, whatever is lovely, whatever is commendable, if there is any excellence, if there is anything worthy of praise, think about these things.*

Proverbs 4:25-27 – *Let your eyes look straight ahead ... Do not swerve to the right or the left.*

Day 19 - PARTNERSHIPS

Ecclesiastes 4:9-12 – *Two are better than one because they have a good reward for their toil. For if they fall, one will lift up his fellow. But woe to him who is alone when he falls and has not another to lift him up! Again, if two lie together, they keep warm, but how can one keep warm alone? And though a man might prevail against one who is alone, two will withstand him—a threefold cord is not quickly broken.*

Proverbs 27:17 – *Iron sharpens iron, and one man sharpens another.*

Matthew 18:20 – *For where two or three are gathered in my name, there am I among them.*

Day 20 - PRIORITIZING

Matthew 6:33 – *But seek first the kingdom of God and his righteousness, and all these things will be added to you.*

Ecclesiastes 10:2 – *The heart of the wise inclines to the right, but the heart of the fool to the left.*

Matthew 6:21 – *For where your treasure is, there your heart will be also.*

3 John 1:2 – *Beloved, I pray that all may go well with you and that you may be in good health, as it goes well with your soul.*

Day 21 – STAYING ON TRACK

James 2:18 – *But someone will say, "You have faith and I have works." Show me your faith apart from your works, and I will show you my faith by my works.*

Proverbs 14:12 – *There is a way that seems right to a man, but its end is the way to death.*

Psalm 119:105 – *Your word is a lamp to my feet and a light to my path.*

S.M.A.R.T. GOAL SETTING

SPECIFIC.

Be specific about the results you want and what you will do to achieve the goal. The Bible offers a very balanced approach to goal-setting. Luke 14:28 teaches us that we need to be specific about our plans and intentions but making sure that they are based on a solid foundation which is in Christ.

You goal outlines the steps it took to arrive at your vision. Remember this: 'fuzzy goals equal fuzzy results'.

Here are some examples of incorrect (non-specific) goals and correct (specific goals):

Not specific: I want to lose some weight.

Specific: I will release 50 pounds by December 31 by starting an exercise program, developing a healthy eating plan, and by allowing the Holy Spirit to guide my food choices.

Not specific: I want to feel better.

Specific: I will participate in the Rock 'n Roll 5k race on May 10, 20XX.

Not specific: I want to have more energy.

Specific: By December 1st, I will have enough energy to be able to climb 20 flights of stairs. I will start with one flight and increase by one flight every week for the next 20 weeks.

The second principle is MEASURABLE. Can you tangibly show how you will meet your goal? What are the objective markers along the way that will confirm that you are moving in the right direction?

You must be able to track your progress to make sure you're on the right track. As one saying goes, 'If you can't measure it, you can't manage it'. Your goals should be able to identify how much, how often, how long, how many, and how you will know when you've reached your goal.

Unfortunately most of us only focus on the scale to measure our progress. This can be very discouraging because it doesn't show the mental changes that are happening in your mind, the spiritual shifts that are breaking strongholds, or the physiological changes that are happening when you burn fat and build muscle.

In Luke 14:28-30 we learn that you would never consider building a house without estimating the costs, the time, and all the factors involved in the project. In the same vein, you would never attempt to start a weight releasing program without having specific indices to measure your success.

Here are some examples of incorrect (non-measurable) goals and correct (measurable goals):

Not measurable: I want to get in better shape.

Measurable: I want to have a BMI of 24, and a body fat percentage of 28%. I want my blood pressure to be 125/85. I want to be able to run five miles without stopping.

In this case you're able to measure your BMI, body fat, and blood pressure. These measurements can be taken weekly and tracked in a journal.

Not measurable: I want to eat healthy foods.

Measurable: I will consume 1500 calories per day consisting of 30% carbohydrates, 35% proteins, and 35% fats.

Setting Attainable Goals

Now it's time to get real about what is and isn't possible. Despite knowing that we'll never achieve this goal, part of us wants to aspire to having our high school body. Or worse yet, if we never had a body that we liked in high school we set out to achieve it anyway, knowing that it's not attainable. Truth is, there are certain things about yourself that you may not ever be able to change no matter how hard you try. If your mother, aunts, grandmothers, great-grandmothers all had wide hips, chances are that you will never look like Gwyneth Paltrow or Taylor Swift no matter how hard you try. Here's where aligning your goals with the Word of God will really come into play. God will show you what *is* possible for you. Have you ever thought about asking Him to show you how much you should weigh? Go ahead, ask Him by writing the question in a journal and then listen for an answer during your quiet time with Him. He may or may not tell you a specific number, but He *will* lead you to a better understanding of what an attainable goal should be for you.

Some women have told me that He has given them an exact number, and some women just remember a time when they felt healthiest and happiest and go with that number.

When thinking about what's attainable for you, consider the following:

1. **Your body type.**

Certain body types are predisposed to 1. carry more weight, or 2. carry weight in certain parts of their body. It's important to understand your body type when deciding a goal weight.

2. **Your commitment level.**

Let's face it, there are no short-cuts or quick fixes to achieving your healthy weight. You've got to commit for the long haul. It might take you six months but for most women it's taken 1-3 years to achieve their goal. Are you willing to commit for that period of time? Before you get frustrated, ask yourself how long it took you to put on the weight. Your success will be directly correlated to your level of commitment.

3. **Your past history with weight loss.**

If you have a history of gaining and losing weight, then there's something significant that you don't know. It will take a lot of unlearning and relearning, which take time. Habits are easy to change, it's the mind that needs convincing.

Next, if you've been dieting on and off for most of your life then your metabolism might be shot—meaning it's not functioning optimally. So your goal may not be attainable until you get your metabolism functioning optimally.

4. **Your trust in God.**

At the end of the day your obedience, which is determined by your level of trust, will be a big determining factor in whether you achieve your goal or not. Despite knowing God is real and

His promises are 'yes' and 'amen', (2 Cor. 1:20) we still struggle with believing Him at His word.

Here's an example of a non-attainable goal:

- Decreasing your hips to 24 inches while increasing your chest size to 38C

Here's an example of setting an attainable goal:

- Attaining a healthy BMI of 24 and waist to hip ratio of .75

In this example, you have to work with what you have. You cannot choose which areas you will take fat from while adding to other areas. Fat is lost usually from the areas where you last gained it. It is also based on your frame, which is God-given. If you've never had large breasts then you probably never will.

Non-attainable goal: wanting to weigh 125 pounds at 50 years old when you're 5'10 and weigh 300 pounds

Attainable:

- achieving a healthy weight of 165-170 pounds

In this example, it can be equally unhealthy to be underweight. If you are tall then you can 'afford' to carry a bit more weight. Wanting to be too thin will not be healthy for you.

"For I know the plans I have for you," declares the LORD. *"Plans to prosper you and not to harm you, plans to give you hope and a future."* (Jeremiah 29:11)

Setting Realistic and Relevant Goals

In order to set realistic goals, you will need to develop an understanding of just what it takes to release weight. Most of our goals are unrealistic because we don't understand the process of weight loss.

Are your goals in line with your Christian values and based on something possible based on your current lifestyle? What may be realistic/relevant for someone else may open the door to sin for you if it takes you to a level of extreme. What may be right for the rest of the world may not be the right thing for you as a believer. Pray and ask for wisdom when you create your goals.

Here are examples of unrealistic goals:

- I will only eat 800 calories per day until I lose the weight.
- I will never eat sweets again.
- I will go to the gym every day for two hours.

Here are examples of realistic goals:

- I will eat 1500 calories per day.
- I will walk for 30 minutes per day.
- I will eat healthy 80% of the time.

Here are examples of irrelevant goals:

- I will have my stomach stapled so I stop overeating.

- I will continue to follow the latest diet.

Here are examples of relevant goals:

- I will weigh what God wants me to weigh by learning what His plan is for my health.
- I will create a healthy meal plan based on what my body needs and choose an exercise that makes my body feel good.

Setting Time-Bound Goals

Time-bound goals mean that your goal should have a start date and an end date. The amount of time that you give yourself to attain your goal should create a sense of urgency, yet should also be realistic enough that it's possible to achieve it. Your mind will adjust accordingly to the deadlines that you set for yourself to accomplish. No timeline means little or no accomplishment.

If you've ever said to yourself, I can't believe that I'm still here, or "I can't believe that I'm still struggling with this same issue", then you know that days, months, years and even decades can quickly pass and you can still find yourself in the same place.

There are a few simple ways to calculate how long it will take you to achieve your goal. Remember, these calculations assume that you're doing what you committed to do at least 80% of the time.

1. The least technical approach is to assume how long it will take you to reach your goal and then double (or triple)that number. That's because most of us underestimate how much we actually eat and over-estimate how much activity we do each day, so this is a simple way to manage your expectations.

2. Assume a half to one pound of weight loss per week and then add an additional three months for holi-days, vacations, illnesses, etc. Choose a half pound if your body doesn't release weight easily and one pound if you're focused. Understand that this formula will only work if you're committed and staying on task.

3. Tracking app. Using a tracking app such as myfit-nesspal or loseit is the best way to more accurately determine how long it will take you to reach your goal. It takes into account your current weight, height, activity level, daily calories consumed, and your resting basal metabolic rate BMR— which is the rate at which your body burns calories at rest.

> *"Therefore be careful how you walk, not as unwise men, but as wise, making the most of your time, because the days are evil."* (Ephesians 5:15, 16)

Putting an end date on your goal does a number of things:

- it creates a sense of urgency
- it helps you to create realistic timelines to work towards
- it will keep you motivated

- it will give you a realistic sense of the amount of effort you need put in to achieve our goal
- it will help you manage and schedule your time

"So teach us to number our days that we may get a heart of wisdom." (Psalm 90:12)

So now that you've learned the S.MA.R.T Principle, let's start to write out your goal.

Write out your goal based on the above.

Here are a few examples:

I, ______________________________, will release 50 pounds (kgs./stones) by February 15, 20XX by releasing two pounds per month. I will do this by learning what foods are right for my body and cutting my calories by 250 per day. I will exercise at least six days per week for 30 minutes and I will learn to see myself the way God sees me.

I, ______________________________, will release 100 pounds (kgs./stones) by June 20XX by releasing five pounds per month. I will join a walking club and walk for one hour per day and add weight training to my workout. I will also track my food on myfitnesspal and maintain my calories at 1400 per day. I will spend time in prayer each morning and ask God to order my steps.

Other Healthy by Design Offerings

Healthy by Design (healthybydesignprogram.com) equips women to rely on God as their strength so they can live in freedom, joy, and peace. At the end of the day, that's what we really want. Let's be honest, if you never achieved that mythical, illusive number on the scale, but were fully able to live a life of freedom, joy, and peace, would that be enough? I know for me the answer is a resounding 'YES!!!'

We provide a multidimensional approach to releasing weight. It encompasses the whole person—spiritual, psychological, mental, nutritional, physical, and even hormonal! We believe that you must address the whole person—body, soul, and spirit. If you're looking for a program that just tells you what to eat and what exercises to do, this ain't it.

This program has helped thousands of women break free from all the roadblocks that have been hindering their weight loss success while discovering their identity in Christ.

Healthy by Design offers a variety of free and paid courses and programs. They include the following:

A YouVersion Bible Study

A free basic introduction to Step 1 of the WLGW program. To learn more, go to:

https://my.bible.com/reading-plans/4593-weight-loss-gods-way.com

Or from the YouVersion Bible App, click the bottom center, 'check-mark' button to open devotions, and search for 'Weight Loss God's Way or our other free devotionals:

Rest, Restore, and Rejuvenate

Praying for Your Health

The Weight Loss, God's Way Newsletter

Join the free *Weight Loss, God's Way* community and receive weekly posts designed to help you align your weight loss with God's Word. You'll also receive our Love Letters from God free download. To join the newsletter, sign up at:

lovegodloseweightbonus.com

The Membership Program

A done-for-you, step-by-step guide to the entire program. Dozens of bonus tools like group coaching calls, forums, and accountability groups. To become a *Weight Loss, God's Way* member, go to:

christianweightlossgodsway.com

Bible Studies for Churches and Small Groups

The membership program can also be experienced a la carte with a group of your friends or with your church. Take one of our three—to-six-week studies on a variety of health and weight-releasing topics. To learn more about starting a Bible study in your home or church, go to:

https://www.cathymorenzie.com/start-a-wlgw-group/

Books and Devotionals

You can find all of our *Healthy by Design* series of weight loss books here:

Christianweightlossbooks.com

Keynote Speaking

Want me to visit your hometown? Need a speaker for your annual conference or special event? My fun and practical approach to *Weight Loss, God's Way* will give your group clarity and focus to move toward their weight loss goals. To learn more or to book a speaking engagement, visit:

https://www.cathymorenzie.com/speaking/

Private Coaching

Prefer a more one-on-one approach? I have a few dedicated time slots available to coach you individually to help you fast-track your results. To learn more, go to:

https://www.cathymorenzie.com/coach-with-cathy-2/

Other Healthy by Design books by Cathy Morenzie:

Healthy Eating, God's Way: 21-Day Meal Plan

Pray Powerfully, Lose Weight

Love God, Lose Weight

Coming soon:

Breakthrough

Strong Faith, Strong Finish

Sugar-Free & Spirit-Filled: 40-Day Detox

Online programs by Cathy Morenzie:

Weight Loss, God's Way 21-Day Challenge:
21daysgodsway.com

5 Steps to Christian Weight Loss Course:
5stepscourse.com

Weight Loss, God's Way Membership:
christianweightlossgodsway.com

Love God, Lose Weight
lovegodloseweight.com

Strong Faith, Strong Finish
strongfaithstrongfinish.com

Pray Powerfully, Lose Weight
praypowerfullyloseweight.com

About The Author

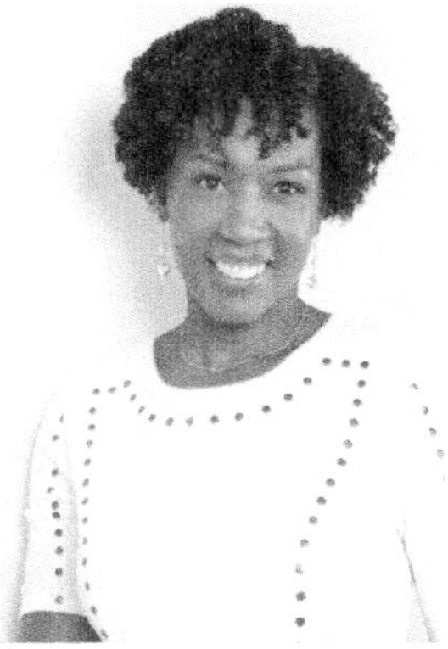

Cathy is a noted personal trainer, author, blogger and presenter, and has been a leader in the faith/fitness industry for over a decade. Her impact has influenced thousands of people over the years to help them lose weight and develop positive attitudes about their bodies and fitness. Over the years, she has seen some of the most powerful and faith-filled people struggle with their health and their weight.

Cathy Morenzie herself—a rational, disciplined, faith-filled personal trainer—struggled with her own weight, emotional eating, self-doubt, and low self-esteem. She tried to change just about everything about herself for much of her life, so she knows what it's like to feel stuck. Every insecurity, challenge, and negative emotion that she experienced has equipped her to help other people who face the same struggles—especially women.

With her Healthy by Design books and Weight Loss, God's Way programs, Cathy has helped thousands to learn to let go of their mental, emotional, and spiritual bonds that have kept them stuck, and instead rely on their Heavenly Father for true release from their fears, doubts, stress, and anxiety. She also teaches people how to eat a sustainable, nutritious diet, and find the motivation to exercise.

Learn more at www.cathymorenzie.com.

Follow Cathy at:
https://www.facebook.com/weightlossgodsway/
https://www.youtube.com/user/activeimage1

Made in the USA
Monee, IL
12 September 2022

13815421R00098